Health Schemes, Scams, and Frauds

Health Schemes, Scams, and Frauds

Stephen Barrett, M.D.,
and the Editors of
Consumer Reports

Consumers Union
Mount Vernon, New York

The information contained in this book is not intended to substitute for professional or medical advice. Consumers Union disclaims responsibility or liability for any loss that may be incurred as a result of the use or application of any information included in *Health Schemes, Scams, and Frauds.* Readers should always consult their physicians or other professionals for treatment and advice. The editors have exercised meticulous care to ensure the accuracy and timeliness of this book. The information contained herein concerning brand names and product formulations was based on the latest available when we went to press. Readers should keep in mind that product names and formulas may change from time to time.

Library of Congress Cataloging-in-Publication Data
Barrett, Stephen, 1933–
Health schemes, scams, and frauds / Stephen Barrett and the editors of Consumer
Reports Books.
    p.   cm.
Includes bibliographical references and index.
ISBN: 0-89043-330-5
1. Quacks and quackery. 2. Quacks and quackery—United States.
3. Consumer protection—United States.   I. Consumer Reports Books.
II Title.
R730.B37   1990
615.8′56′0973—dc20   90-40919
                                      CIP

Design by GDS / Jeffrey L. Ward
First printing, January 1991
Manufactured in the United States of America

Consumer Reports Books

Health Schemes, Scams, and Frauds is a Consumer Reports Book published by Consumers Union, the nonprofit organization that publishes *Consumer Reports*, the monthly magazine of test reports, product Ratings, and buying guidance. Established in 1936, Consumers Union is chartered under the Not-for-Profit Corporation Law of the State of New York.

The purposes of Consumers Union, as stated in its charter, are to provide consumers with information and counsel on consumer goods and services, to give information on all matters relating to the expenditure of the family income, and to initiate and to cooperate with individual and group efforts seeking to create and maintain decent living standards.

Consumers Union derives its income solely from the sale of *Consumer Reports* and other publications. In addition, expenses of occasional public service efforts may be met, in part, by nonrestrictive, noncommercial contributions, grants, and fees. Consumers Union accepts no advertising or product samples and is not beholden in any way to any commercial interest. Its Ratings and reports are solely for the use of the readers of its publications. Neither the Ratings, nor the reports, nor any Consumers Union publications, including this book, may be used in advertising or for any commercial purpose. Consumers Union will take all steps open to it to prevent such uses of its materials, its name, or the name of *Consumer Reports*.

Contents

Preface

Health Schemes, Scams, and Frauds is based in part on articles originally published in the pages of *Consumer Reports*, the monthly magazine published by Consumers Union. Such material has been extensively rewritten, updated, and expanded with the assistance of Consumers Union's medical consultants. Much of the book contains new, unpublished information researched by Stephen Barrett, M.D.

Dr. Barrett, an award-winning consumer advocate, editor, and author, is a board member of the National Council Against Health Fraud and a scientific and editorial adviser to the American Council on Science and Health. A psychiatrist who practices in Allentown, Pennsylvania, and editor of *Nutrition Forum Newsletter*, he has produced 25 books, including *The Health Robbers, Vitamins and Health Foods—The Great American Hustle,* and the college textbook *Consumer Health—A Guide to Intelligent Decisions.*

1

Health Quackery:
Promising the Impossible

Quackery has existed, said Voltaire, since the first knave met the first fool. Perhaps the eighteenth-century French philosopher had the unicorn in mind. For centuries this one-horned beast, which lived only in human imagination, was believed to be the source of a potent remedy. Indeed, "unicorn horn" was touted for epilepsy, impotence, worms, the plague, smallpox, mad dog bites, and a variety of other complaints.

"In spite of the lack of the actual animal, the horn was usually available—at a price," Wallace C. Ellerbroek, M.D., observed in 1968 in the *Journal of the American Medical Association*. "The value of the horns varied with the supply, and at the peak of the market, the powder and pieces brought up to ten times their weight in gold."

By Voltaire's day, numerous patent medicines were being sold throughout Europe and the American colonies. Typical of that era, Benjamin Franklin's *Pennsylvania Gazette* ran ads for the Widow Read's "Ointment for the Itch," which was supposed to drive away lice as well as "the most inveterate Itch." (The Widow Read was none other than Franklin's mother-in-law.)

Quackery continued to prosper in America. In 1856 a pharmacist reported that scores of nostrums were marketed whose chief mission appeared to be "to open men's purses by opening their bowels." At that time, medical treatment—which included bloodletting and purging—was often no better and sometimes worse than the remedies of charlatans. But the discoveries of Louis Pasteur, Robert Koch, Joseph Lister, and others touched off the explosive growth of medical science.

Throughout the development of modern medicine, says this country's leading historian of quackery, James Harvey Young, Ph.D., emeritus professor of history at Emory University, "quackery's demise has often been predicted." Writing in 1972, Dr. Young commented that Americans believed themselves to be "a reasonable people, and if error persisted here and there, it would soon vanish because of our corporate good sense. . . . When the populace had received a little more public schooling, when science had expanded its horizons a little further, or when Congress had enacted such-and-such a protective law, then would quackery vanish, consigned to the museum of outmoded delusions."

But, to paraphrase Mark Twain, the reports of quackery's imminent death were greatly exaggerated. In fact, it has thrived despite wider opportunities for public education, enormous advances in medical technology, and the passage of laws intended to ensure drug safety and effectiveness and protect against fraud in the health marketplace.

According to the U.S. Food and Drug Administration (FDA), the term *quackery* encompasses both people and products: the health practitioner who has a "miracle cure" but no medical training is a quack (even a medical degree offers no

guarantee against fraudulent practices); the drug or food supplement promoted with false health claims is a quack product:
and the machine that has impressive knobs and dials but does
nothing except take money out of the pockets of the unsuspecting is a quack device. Broadly speaking, says the FDA,
"quackery is the promotion of a medical remedy that doesn't
work or hasn't been proven to work."

Today, quackery is a multibillion-dollar business, but the
money wasted each year on quack products and services is
only part of the problem. No one knows how many people
have died of cancer because they relied on quack treatment
until it was too late for conventional therapy to be of help.
Or how many arthritis victims have dissipated their life savings
chasing false hopes—while their disease and disability grew
worse.

In 1984, the late Claude Pepper, chairman of the House
Select Committee on Aging's Subcommittee on Health and
Long-Term Care, released a 250-page summary of what he
called "the most comprehensive review of quackery ever undertaken by a Congressional body." Based on a four-year investigation, the report concluded:

> Quackery has traveled far from the day of the pitch-
> man and covered wagon to emerge as big business.
> Those who orchestrate and profit from the sale and
> promotion of these useless and often harmful
> "health" products are no longer quaint and comical
> figures. They are well organized, sophisticated, and
> persistent.

Here in the 1990s, they're still going strong.

Vulnerability to Quackery

Some of quackery's hardy nostrums—bust developers, bald-ness remedies, "anti-aging" products, weight-loss aids that "melt away" fat without dieting—are hawked largely through mail-order advertisements. But many quack schemes and products are promoted more subtly: in books, in magazine and newspaper articles, on radio and television talk shows, at "health food" expos, in the halls of Congress by skillful lob-byists—and occasionally by legislators themselves. And "nu-tritional" methods touted by self-appointed experts and dissident physicians can deceive otherwise knowledgeable in-dividuals as deftly as ads for bust developers or hair restorers can fool the naive.

Despite Voltaire's dictum, quackery has never been limited to transactions between knaves and fools. Indeed, its victims come from all walks of life and educational backgrounds. As noted by Dr. Young, "few escape blindspots and areas of error that make them vulnerable to quackery under suitable cir-cumstances. This goes for some of mighty intellect with var-ious degrees after their names."

Nor is the promotion of quackery limited to people who lack scientific training. A small but significant percentage of well-trained individuals have strayed into providing unproven and irrational therapies—even for diseases as serious as cancer and heart disease. Some also offer unjustified diagnoses with "treatments" to match.

Nor does quackery always involve fraudulent intent. "Whether from self-delusion, insanity, or simple ignorance, many quacks are sincerely dedicated to their nostrums," says William T. Jarvis, Ph.D., professor of preventive medicine at Loma Linda University and president of the National Council

Against Health Fraud. "Some have actually killed themselves or their loved ones with their favorite remedies."

Perhaps the trickiest misconception about quackery is the belief that personal experience is the best way to tell whether something works. When someone feels better after having used a product or procedure, it seems natural to give credit to whatever was done. Such faith in anecdotal experiences may be blind. Most ailments are self-limiting, and even incurable conditions can have sufficient day-to-day or week-to-week variation to enable quack methods to gain large followings. In addition, the very act of doing something may produce temporary relief of symptoms. The placebo effect is a force to be reckoned with. Any attention, medication, or procedure, even if shown to be ineffective, may improve a person's symptoms. For these reasons, scientific experimentation is almost always necessary to establish whether health methods are really effective.

The extent to which people can be fooled should not be underestimated. According to an article by FDA historian Wallace Janssen in the *FDA Consumer*, during the 1930s and 1940s thousands became convinced that "Glyoxylide," a remedy promoted by William Koch, M.D., Ph.D., could cure cancer. More than 3,000 health practitioners of various kinds paid $25 per ampule and charged patients up to $300 for a single injection. Yet analysis of the product showed it to be distilled water!

Quacks Never Sleep

"Down through the ages," Dr. Jarvis says, "people have sought four types of 'magic potions': the fountain of youth, the love potion, the cure-all, and the athletic superpill. Quackery has always been willing to cater to these desires."

Sure enough, quacks and quackery keep up with the times. The graying of our population has spawned a host of "anti-aging" products for the prevention and treatment of degenerative diseases. The fitness boom has fostered a multitude of bogus products claiming to enhance athletic ability. Concerns about diet and disease have inspired many food companies to make claims that go beyond what is scientifically proven. But no category of quackery has mushroomed more quickly in modern times than the realm of AIDS-related products.

AIDS (acquired immunodeficiency syndrome) is caused by a virus that disrupts the body's immune system, rendering it unable to resist certain infections and some forms of cancer. Since no cure for AIDS exists, reputable physicians can only delay the onset of those opportunistic diseases that take advantage of the victim's damaged immune system. Once infections become recurrent, antibiotic treatment becomes increasingly ineffective. But quackery promises more. Experts who have surveyed the marketplace have concluded that "almost everything is being converted into an AIDS treatment." More than 200 bogus treatments have been reported, and many of the clinics offering dubious cancer treatments now claim their approach also works against AIDS.

During 1987 John Renner, M.D., a board member of the National Council Against Health Fraud, visited more than 30 health food stores and attended four "health expos" sponsored by groups that promote unorthodox remedies. When he inquired about products for AIDS, he was offered processed blue-green algae (pond scum) selling for $20 a bottle, injectable hydrogen peroxide, garlic "to boost the immune system," pills said to have been derived from mice that had been given the AIDS virus, BHT (a food preservative), and herbal capsules that later were found to contain poisonous metals—all irrational nostrums. Other "treatments" he encountered included bathing the body in a chlorine bleach solution and thumping on the thymus gland.

The AIDS marketplace is by no means limited to people who already have the disease. Fear of catching it has created a much wider potential market for "preventive" measures. Health food-industry manufacturers have formulated vitamin/mineral/amino acid concoctions claimed to "strengthen the immune system." A few companies have marketed telephone mouthpiece covers and similar products claimed to prevent transmission of the AIDs virus through public facilities—not even a theoretical mode of transmission since the virus dies quickly when exposed to ordinary surfaces. Some firms have illegally marketed AIDS test kits since none has been approved by the FDA. Some dating services tout an "AIDS-free" clientele, even though it is impossible to monitor the sexual contacts of each and every client—nor would they be able to tell when someone who tests negative is incubating the disease.

In 1989 the Houston-based Consumer Health Education Council surveyed 41 health food stores. To collect the data, council members said that they had a brother with AIDS who was having intolerable side effects with a prescribed drug (AZT) and that the brother's wife wanted to keep from becoming infected while having sex with him. Nicolas Martin, the council's executive director, reported:

> Every one of the stores offered to sell us one product or another for the disease or its symptoms. They were also anxious to load us down with supplements which were claimed to prevent or make it harder for

an uninfected person to catch AIDS. Not one mentioned something simple like using condoms. Many told us that while the AIDS virus could not be eliminated from the body it could be "suppressed," or "deactivated" so that all symptoms would disappear. Others told us flatly that AIDs could be cured using whatever they recommended.

Consumer Protection: Limited

The FDA can take action when a food, drug, cosmetic, or medical device sold in interstate commerce is misbranded or includes false or misleading claims in its labeling (which includes accompanying literature and point-of-sale advertising). The agency can also act against such products if they are dangerous or, in the case of drugs, ineffective, and against products that are sold before complying with certain premarket requirements. When wrongdoing is detected, the FDA can seek voluntary correction, have the product seized, obtain an injunction, or initiate criminal prosecution against the offender. However, criminal prosecution is rarely used in quackery cases.

The interstate commerce requirement also applies to the Federal Trade Commission (FTC), which is empowered to act against false and misleading advertising of health services or products (except for prescription drugs, which are under FDA jurisdiction). The FTC can also issue regulations and seek injunctions to halt unfair or deceptive trade practices. Although FTC action can result in a large financial penalty, the agency usually handles only five or six cases per year involving health frauds.

A third federal agency, the U.S. Postal Service, can take

action against anyone—including a purveyor of quack products—who uses the mail to defraud. When a scam is detected, postal officials can take administrative action to obtain a cease-and-desist order and to block mail containing money or product orders from reaching the perpetrator. Recent changes in the law have increased the Postal Service's ability to deal with mail-order quackery—making it possible to seek large fines against repeat offenders.

One might suppose that the three agencies together could do a reasonably good job of policing quackery. Each of them, however, has a relatively circumscribed area of authority, and a relatively small staff, with a heavy load of other responsibilities. It also can be difficult to stop a determined peddler of questionable health products or services. The FDA spent more than a decade in the courts before the worthless Hoxsey cancer clinics closed down, and a similar period struggling to ban Laetrile. In another classic case, it took 16 years of litigation, with 11,000 pages of testimony and 150 exhibits, for the FTC to get the word *Liver* removed from "Carter's Little Liver Pills."

Even when all three agencies attack the same company, they may not succeed in stopping its illegal activity unless the attack is relentless. The most noteworthy example of this situation is General Nutrition Corporation (GNC), which operates the nation's largest chain of health food stores and, until recently, owned a mail-order division carrying most of the same products. In 1985 the company signed consent agreements with the Postal Service to stop making unsubstantiated claims for 14 products sold through the mail. In 1986 an administrative-law judge in the FTC ruled that GNC ads for an alleged cancer preventative were deliberately misleading and concluded that the "unconscionable, false, and misleading advertising found in this case is not an isolated incident but part of a continuing pattern." The same year, to settle criminal charges initiated by the FDA, the company pleaded guilty to four counts of misbranding a drug, and its former president and another officer pleaded guilty to one count. In 1988 the FTC complaint was settled by a consent agreement in which GNC agreed to donate $600,000 for nutrition research and was prohibited from making any claim for any company-produced product that cannot be substantiated by scientific evidence.

As a result of these actions, various products were discontinued, but GNC's mail-order division (sold in 1989 to Nature's Bounty, Incorporated, of Bohemia, New York) continues to violate the law. At the request of an FTC attorney, a medical consultant for Consumers Union (CU) analyzed the February 1990 catalog and found 42 products that either are unapproved new drugs or are advertised with false and/or misleading claims.

Although a few states have aggressive antiquackery programs, most state and local enforcement agencies are so poorly staffed that they can act only infrequently against health frauds; and when they do, the offender may merely pay a fine—and move the operation elsewhere.

Health professionals are regulated by state licensing boards, which can take action against unprofessional conduct. However, most of these agencies have shown little interest in trying to curb quack practices. Even when a state board takes action, a determined practitioner may be able to continue practicing for years while appealing the board's ruling through the courts.

Since government action against quackery is limited, individuals wishing to protect themselves must be vigilant. With this book, CU seeks to spotlight the most prevalent and persistent forms of quackery. The following chapters explore the promotion of worthless remedies for cancer and arthritis, the false claims made for chiropractic treatments, homeopathic remedies, and weight-reducing schemes, the scare campaigns against mercury-amalgam ("silver") fillings, the overselling of vitamins and other "food supplements," the misrepresentation of hypogylcemia and candidiasis hypersensitivity as widespread diseases, the use of mail-order schemes to defraud consumers, and other dubious products and practices in the health marketplace. These chapters also suggest ways to reduce quackery's toll on society.

2

Facts Versus Fictions

Years ago, some surgeons thought they had developed a promising cure for angina pectoris, the chest pains associated with coronary heart disease. By tying off a branch of an artery inside the chest they hoped to divert more blood to the heart, and apparently it worked. But the popularity of the procedure was short-lived. Subsequent research showed that a sham operation, consisting of just a superficial incision on the chest wall, was equally successful at relieving anginal pain.

The experiment, albeit somewhat extreme, demonstrates the broad influence of the "placebo effect," a reaction to an inactive preparation or procedure associated with improvement or cure of symptoms. (Placebos can also produce undesirable side effects.) It matters little whether the treatment takes the form of surgery, drugs, food supplements, manipulation, incantations, or something else. Confidence in the treatment—on the part of the patient and the practitioner—makes it more likely that a positive effect will occur. But even a suggestible nonbeliever may respond favorably. The only requirement for a placebo effect is the awareness that something has been done.

Throughout much of medical history, the placebo effect was frequently all any healer could offer. Indeed, it was often fortunate if the actual treatment had some psychological value or perhaps was merely worthless, rather than harmful or fatal. Today, despite all the knowledge and paraphernalia of modern medicine, such psychological effects are still an important factor in therapy. They account for some of the benefits obtained by the most skillful physicians. Such effects also explain, in part, why unscientific practices can appear to help people. In many disorders 30 to 40 percent of patients will show improvement with use of a placebo. Temporary relief has been demonstrated, for example, in arthritis, hay fever, headache, cough, high blood pressure, premenstrual tension, peptic ulcer, and even cancer. Psychological aspects of many disorders also work to the healer's advantage. A sizable percentage of symptoms have a psychological component, and many do not arise from organic disease at all. Hence treatment offering some easing of tension can often help. A sympathetic ear or reassurance that no serious disease is involved may prove therapeutic by itself.

In addition to psychological influences in treatment, the recuperative powers of the body itself must be taken into consideration. As already noted, most human ailments are self-limiting. No matter what type of intervention or treatment is used, most people eventually improve on their own. Even some chronic disorders, such as rheumatoid arthritis and multiple sclerosis, have spontaneous remissions. The symptoms may disappear, regardless of treatment for months or more, affording temporary or, at times, long-term relief. If the patient happens to be under treatment at the time, the practitioner and the type of therapy may get undeserved credit for such relief.

The noted astronomer Carl Sagan has pointed out that "at the heart of science are two seemingly contradictory attitudes—an openness to new ideas, no matter how bizarre they seem, and the most ruthless scrutiny of all ideas, old and new. This is how deep truths are winnowed from deep nonsense." Medical truths can be especially complicated to derive because of the placebo effect and the variability of disease. Thus stringent rules are needed to determine whether a particular drug or procedure is effective—or whether an outcome has another explanation.

The Scientific Method

For more than a century, scientists throughout the world have been following agreed-upon practices to determine how things work. These practices—known collectively as the "scientific method"—are embraced by all fields of science, not just medicine. They include defining the problem, collecting data through careful observation and experimentation, setting up hypotheses, and testing them.

In medical research there are many ways to obtain preliminary data. Epidemiology involves comparing population groups to see whether differences in the incidence of disease can be correlated with other factors. This approach often provides important clues about the possible causes of disease. Valuable information may be obtained from laboratory experiments with animals, tissue cultures, and various test-tube preparations. Studies using small numbers of people can still yield significant data. Controlled studies compare people who receive a treatment with similar subjects getting a placebo. The ultimate test is "double blind": neither the researchers nor the people being tested know who is getting which treatment. Blinding is desirable to ensure that none of the participants allow their personal biases to interfere with accurate observation. Enough people must be used to make it statistically unlikely that the outcome occurs merely by chance. To gain acceptance by scientists, an experiment must be capable of yielding similar results by other researchers.

Gradually, bits and pieces of knowledge may be forged into a consistent framework of ideas. When a study is completed, the researchers strive to publish their results in a medical journal. That way, others can consider and possibly use the findings or criticize them or seek to reproduce them. The best medical journals are peer-reviewed. This means that before being accepted for publication, a study is evaluated by scientists working in the same or a similar field; they help the editors decide whether a paper is worthy of publication or if the authors need to provide additional data. Two of the most respected medical publications are the *Journal of the American Medical Association* and *The New England Journal of Medicine*. Important issues are also addressed by councils and committees that are trusted by the medical community.

These activities can help medical educators and practicing physicians to identify accepted scientific views and conduct their activities accordingly. The participants in this process—basic scientists, clinical researchers, journal editors, educators, and practitioners—are often referred to collectively as the "scientific community." *The judgments in this book are based on what CU considers to be the collective wisdom of the scientific community*. If a theory, practice, or product is not backed by scientific evidence, CU considers it unproven. If it appears

inconsistent with well-established facts, CU may label it unscientific, dubious, or questionable. If it involves deliberate
deception by its proponents, CU may also call it fraudulent.

"Alternative" Notions

Perhaps the main difference between science and pseudoscience is the rigidity of the latter. Science is self-correcting
and expands or revises its belief as new evidence arises. If a
new concept doesn't fit with accepted scientific beliefs, the
scientific community will determine whether the concept is
flawed or current beliefs must be altered. But quack beliefs—
no matter how illogical they are or how often they are re-
futed—are rarely abandoned by their promoters as long as
they are marketable.

The procedures described above have enabled medical science to make remarkable progress. But some unscientific practitioners described in this book view things differently. They
suggest that disease has one basic cause—a failure of the body
to protect itself—which can be corrected by whatever they
happen to believe. Fringe medical practitioners, for example,
typically allege that allergies or metabolic imbalances are the
underlying cause of innumerable symptoms. "Natural health"
advocates claim that the main causes of ill health are "pollution" and faulty living habits. When health fails, they say,
the way to restore it is to conform to "nature's laws" through
dietary improvement, exercise, and various measures to "detoxify" the body. Taking conventional drugs merely exposes
the body to further pollution.

Some unscientific approaches are based on the magical idea
that an object of enchantment can be "mapped" onto an accessible place and manipulated to control one's destiny. Thus,

while chiropractors concentrate on the spine, acupuncturists needle the skin, reflexologists massage the hands or feet, and iridologists focus on the eyes. The effects they claim may not be demonstrable by scientific tests, but so what? Since satisfied customers attest to the correctness of their approach, further proof is unnecessary.

Many unscientific promoters claim that their methods are effective not only for treating disease but also for preventing it—which enables them to fleece healthy people as well as sick people.

Unscientific practitioners often claim that they are "too busy helping sick people get well" to demonstrate the efficacy of their treatment by performing research acceptable to the scientific community. This is a ploy. It is neither time-consuming nor expensive to conduct a simple follow-up study in which the condition of patients before and after treatment is carefully documented. In fact, most of the data needed for such a study should be recorded as part of ordinary medical practice. If an unproven treatment for a serious disease really shows promise, independent researchers will be eager to evaluate it.

Advertising Hype

Whereas pseudoscientists typically dismiss the results of scientific studies, advertisers may embellish or distort the meaning of such studies. For example, claims may be based on studies that are poorly designed or are unconfirmed; on reports whose conclusions are taken out of context; or on animal experiments not necessarily applicable to humans.

In 1982 the National Academy of Sciences (NAS) reported that the incidence of certain cancers might be reduced by eating a diet rich in fruits and vegetables, particularly those high in vitamin C and beta-carotene (which the body can convert into vitamin A). The report emphasized that since it was not known which dietary factors, if any, might be helpful, supplementation with individual nutrients is not advisable. Despite this caveat, several companies began marketing tablets containing dehydrated vegetables and various nutrients mentioned in the NAS report. Ads for these products even suggested that the report had advocated their use.

Since the ads were clearly fraudulent, the FTC was able to drive these products from the marketplace. But beta-carotene capsules are still marketed with a more subtle approach. Some manufacturers have mentioned the NAS report and suggested that if you aren't eating foods rich in beta-carotene, supplementation might make sense. Others simply describe how beta-carotene supplementation is being studied as a possible cancer preventative. Readers of the ads are encouraged to think about beta-carotene and calculate those odds for themselves.

The recent public focus on the relationship between diet and heart disease has spawned an enormous number of related advertising claims. It is well established that elevated blood cholesterol is a risk factor for coronary artery disease and that, for most people, the amount of saturated fat in the diet is a major factor influencing the blood cholesterol level. Dietary cholesterol can also play a role, but not nearly as much. For this reason, people wishing to lower their blood cholesterol level through dietary means should be much more concerned with the amount of saturated fat they consume than the amount of cholesterol.

Unfortunately, since the public is much more familiar with "cholesterol" than with "saturated fat," many manufacturers have been making "no-cholesterol" claims even for foods high in saturated fat. Thus unsuspecting consumers interested in trying to adopt healthier eating habits might actually make things worse by eating these "no cholesterol" foods. The FDA has proposed regulations dealing with this problem but has moved so slowly that the marketplace has become chaotic.

The March 1990 issue of *Consumer Reports* contained a report on the cholesterol issue and on the growing practice of advertisers to use disease-prevention claims to sell foods. In particular, some entrepreneurs are marketing "cholesterol-lowering" nostrums. These products typically contain niacin, oat bran, fish oil, lecithin, garlic, and various other substances. Niacin can play an important role in a medically supervised cholesterol-reducing program, but the amounts in these products are too small to be effective—as are the amounts of oat bran. Fish oils are effective only in high doses, which can have serious side effects. Lecithin, garlic, and the rest have no proven role in lowering blood cholesterol.

Of course, the advertising claims for some health products—particularly those sold by mail—are complete fabrications.

How Consumers Can Protect Themselves

How can health facts be separated from health fictions? How can the consumer judge who is trustworthy? These questions are crucial because wrong answers can be harmful to health as well as expensive. The best approach is to maintain a reasonable level of skepticism, learn the typical signs of unscientific thought, and choose sources of information carefully.

3

Fringe Medicine

"How is your thirst?" he asks the patient, a woman who is in for her first visit. "Do you drink a whole glass of water at a time or just sip it?

"Do you drink tap water? Ice water?

"Do you eat ice?

"Do you like your home temperature warm or cold?"

The questioner, whose manner is friendly and alert, is David Wember, M.D., of Falls Church, Virginia. His office resembles that of a typical family practitioner, except for the cabinets and open shelves containing thousands of remedies in small bottles. For more than a decade, he has practiced homeopathy, a form of medicine popular in the 1800s. Homeopaths believe that extremely tiny doses of the proper substance will stimulate the body's natural defenses against an illness.

While a physician on assignment as a CU reporter was present in 1986, Dr. Wember saw patients for headaches, diarrhea, obesity, chronic tension, and arthritis—complaints typical for any general medical office. On most workdays, he sees 10 to 12 patients, new ones for an hour and others for a half-hour—"a bit more time than the average medical doctor"—he pointed out. Each patient is asked standard medical questions plus many more involving emotions, moods, food preferences, and reactions to the weather.

"Homeopathy is based on all of the patient's symptoms, both emotional and physical," Dr. Wember explained. "This includes likes and dislikes, cravings and aversions to foods, and the patient's relationship to the environment."

When a familiar pattern emerges from a patient's answers, Dr. Wember checks his reference book on homeopathic medicines and asks further questions to confirm his hunch. The remedy arrived at, he removes a few granules from one of his many bottles, places the substance on the patient's tongue, and arranges for another appointment. Sometimes he prescribes conventional drugs, but he usually favors starting with homeopathic remedies.

Inquiries about food preferences or minor personal idiosyncrasies seldom play a part in conventional medical diagnosis. But no competent physician of any stripe would argue against the importance of taking a careful medical history. Where homeopaths and orthodox physicians part company is in the type of remedies they prescribe—and in the rationales behind these two contrasting approaches to medical treatment.

Like Cures Like

Homeopathy is the brainchild of Samuel Hahnemann, a German physician who formulated its principles in the late 1700s. Hahnemann was distressed by the medical practices of his day, which included extensive bloodletting, purging, blistering, and large, or "heroic," doses of medicine. He soon abandoned such treatment and started prescribing exercise, fresh air, and a nourishing diet. He also began experimenting with drugs, commonly taking the medicine himself and recording its effects.

An early experiment involved quinine, which was already in use for treating malaria. Hahnemann doubted the prevailing theory that the bitter drug cured malaria by the "strengthening qualities" it exerted on the stomach. When he took it, he experienced thirst, throbbing in the head, and fever—symptoms common to malaria. He decided that the drug's power to cure the disease arose from its ability to produce symptoms similar to the disease itself.

Such experiments, which Hahnemann called "provings," led to his first principle of homeopathy—the "Law of Similars," or "like cures like." Hahnemann and his early followers conducted many such provings. They administered herbs, minerals, and other substances to healthy people, including themselves, and recorded what they observed. Later, these records were compiled into reference books called *materia medica*, which are used to match a patient's symptoms with a corresponding drug.

Less Is More

Hahnemann also believed that disease represents a disturbance in the body's ability to heal itself, and that only a small stimulus is needed to start the healing process. In keeping with this theory—and to avoid toxic side effects—Hahnemann experimented to see how little medication might still produce a healing response. Eventually he concluded that the smaller the dose, the more powerful the effect.

Pharmacologists today conclude exactly the opposite: the larger the dose, the greater the effect. But current homeopathic remedies are still based on Hahnemann's nineteenth-century theory. They are prepared by repeatedly diluting the active ingredient until only a minuscule dose remains. Dilutions are commonly made by factors of 10, indicated on the product by multiples of the Roman numeral X. Thus 1X means a 10-fold dilution, 2X is 100-fold, 3X is 1,000-fold, and so on. Most dosages today range from 6X—one part per million—to 30X. If dilutions are made by factors of 100, the Roman numeral C is used instead.

According to the laws of chemistry, there's a limit to how much diluting can occur without losing the original substance altogether. This limit, called Avogadro's number, corresponds closely to the homeopathic dosage 24X. Hahnemann realized it was unlikely that even a single molecule of the original substance would remain after such dilution. But he believed that the vigorous shaking or pulverizing with each step of the process left behind a spiritlike essence of the original substance that helped revive the body's "vital force."

Whatever the theory, the watered-down homeopathic medicines were safer than many of the nineteenth century's orthodox drugs, which sometimes posed more of a threat to the patient than the disease. Many of Hahnemann's medical contemporaries began using his remedies, often with better results than they had with orthodox preparations. At least the minute dosages did no harm, allowing patients a fighting chance to recover on their own.

By the mid-1800s, homeopathy had become a prominent alternative to established medicine. The founding of the

American Medical Association in 1846 was in part an attempt to put down this rival faction. But homeopathy survived in force until the end of the century, when it numbered some 14,000 practitioners and 22 schools in the United States alone. However, the advance of science in the twentieth century proved far more potent than the attacks of organized medicine. The development of drugs and other therapies that were clearly effective drove homeopathy into a sharp decline, particularly in the United States. By the 1920s, most of its U.S. schools had closed, and its ranks in this country eventually dwindled to just a few hundred practitioners.

Despite its vestigial state, homeopathy retained some political clout. Its remedies were accorded legal status by the 1938 Federal Food, Drug, and Cosmetic Act, which was shepherded through Congress by a U.S. senator from New York who was also a prominent homeopathic physician.

Unlike most other legal drugs, homeopathic remedies have never been judged effective by the FDA. But a provision of the 1938 law includes within its definition of drugs all substances listed in the *Homeopathic Pharmacopeia of the United States*. The basis of their inclusion is not modern scientific testing but homeopathic "provings" done as long as 150 years ago.

Until the mid-1970s, the FDA remained untroubled by the dubious scientific credentials of homeopathic drugs. Homeopathy appeared to be heading for extinction, and its remedies were expected to vanish with it. Although most of the products are prescription drugs, the FDA tended to look the other way when some occasionally surfaced in the over-the-counter market. The tiny dosages were considered innocuous—the equivalent of a placebo—and traffic in the products appeared meager.

But homeopathy's anticipated demise failed to arrive. In recent years, according to the FDA, the back-to-nature movement and a growing infatuation with all things "natural" have helped breathe new life into the fading practice. Offering a "nonchemical" way of treating illness without side effects, homeopathy has caught the wave of the trend.

Riding the Resurgence

In most states, anyone licensed to prescribe drugs can practice homeopathy. If only licensed practitioners are counted, the resurgence in homeopathy appears modest. The 1990 directory of the National Center for Homeopathy, in Washington, D.C., lists about 350 licensed practitioners, approximately half of them physicians and the rest mostly dentists, veterinarians, nurses, naturopaths, and chiropractors. But a disturbing trend, says the FDA, is that a growing number of unlicensed people are now calling themselves homeopaths and setting up practices to cash in on the revival. The FDA reports that some are using homeopathic drugs, including injectibles, to treat serious diseases.

Also worrisome, says the agency, is a steep rise in over-the-counter sales of homeopathic remedies. William G. Nychis, the FDA's expert on homeopathy, has noted that "the homeopathic marketplace has changed drastically. New firms have entered the field and have been selling all sorts of products through health food stores and directly to consumers."

In a survey conducted back in 1982, the FDA found some over-the-counter products being marketed for serious illnesses, including heart disease, kidney disorders, and cancer. An extract of tarantula was being purveyed for multiple sclerosis, an extract of cobra venom for cancer. Four years later, CU found similar products being sold at health food stores, by mail, and even person-to-person through multilevel marketing companies. Twelve firms offered products with such names as *Circulation Formula*, *Heart Tonic*, *Hepatic Dysfunction Drops*, *Renal Forte*, and the like. As one longtime marketer of homeopathic remedies put it, "There is a lot of insanity operating under the name of homeopathy in today's marketplace."

The revival of homeopathy—in one form or another—has also awakened the FDA to the need to regulate it. But only a few of the most flagrant violators have felt the agency's sting. For example, during 1988 the agency took action against companies marketing "diet patches" with false claims that they could suppress appetite. (The largest such company, Meditrend International, of San Diego, instructed users to place one or two drops of a "homeopathic appetite control solution" on a patch and wear it all day affixed to an "acupuncture point" on the wrist to "bioelectrically" suppress the appetite control center of the brain.) As time goes on, the agency may get around to other violators. Judging by its past performance, though, it's doubtful that the market will be cleaned up soon.

The health food industry is well aware of the unique regulatory status of homeopathic remedies. A recent article in the trade publication *Whole Foods* reported that "there is more freedom in selling homeopathy than most other categories." Another article even suggested that "when a customer comes into your store complaining of an earache, fever, flu, sore throat, diarrhea or some other common health problem . . . one word that should immediately come out of your mouth is 'homeopathy.' "

Ironically, the promotional emphasis on such products runs directly counter to a central concept of homeopathy—the painstaking, individualized attention to a patient's symptoms before prescribing a remedy. That attention, which may relieve the patient's anxiety or produce a placebo effect, may well be the most therapeutic part of classic homeopathy, today as well as in the 1800s.

High-Tech Homeopathy?

A few doctors who consider themselves homeopaths use "electrodiagnostic" machines to aid them in prescribing remedies. Fuller Royal, M.D., director of the Nevada Clinic in Las Vegas, is the main proponent of this method in the United States. Royal has been on Nevada's homeopathic licensing board and was its president from 1983 to 1985.

All patients at his clinic are diagnosed with a machine called the Interro. The computerized device is said to measure changes in the skin's electrical resistance, indicating whether the body's organ systems have proper "electromagnetic energy balance." Using a probe connected to the machine, the doctor touches "acupuncture points" on the patient's hands and feet and interprets numbers that appear on the computer screen. He then uses the machine to select homeopathic remedies that are supposed to correct "imbalances" in energy flow.

Nevada Clinic publications state that electrodiagnosis is one of the most effective ways to diagnose illness. "There are no incurable diseases, only ignorant physicians," say the publications. The first clinic visit, which spans a two-day period, commonly costs $700 to $800, including $165 for allergy testing and $100 for homeopathic remedies.

When CU's physician-reporter visited the Nevada Clinic in 1986, he noticed that the main thing determining what numbers appear on the Interro's screen is how hard the probes are pressed against the patient's fingers or toes. Dr. Royal readily acknowledged this but said, "that's why it takes a lot of training to use the equipment properly."

Nevada's homeopathic licensing law—which Dr. Royal helped design—includes "noninvasive electrodiagnosis" within the definition of homeopathy. When asked whether the electrodiagnostic devices are legal under federal law, an FDA official replied that the agency considered the devices a "significant risk" but was hesitant to act because they are legal under Nevada law. Meanwhile, insurance companies that balk at paying for treatment by Nevada homeopaths have been threatened with sanctions by the state's insurance commissioner.

Dubious Chemistry

Unless the laws of chemistry have gone awry, most homeopathic remedies are too dilute to have any physiological effect. For that reason, medical scientists consider them to be innocuous but absurd drugs. During 1986, for example, faculty members from 49 U.S. pharmacy schools answered a CU questionnaire on homeopathy. Virtually all the respondents said the remedies were neither potent nor effective, except possibly as placebos for mild, temporary ailments that commonly resolve on their own.

Medical consultants for CU believe that any system of medicine embracing the use of such remedies involves a potential danger to patients, whether the prescribers are M.D.s, other licensed practitioners, or outright quacks. Ineffective drugs are dangerous when used to treat serious or life-threatening disease. Moreover, even though homeopathic drugs are essentially nontoxic, self-medication can still be hazardous. Using such remedies for a serious illness or undiagnosed pain instead of obtaining proper medical attention could prove harmful or even fatal.

Public protection regarding drugs is based on a framework of federal laws and regulations, which require that such products be safe, effective, and free of false claims in labeling. The FDA has yet to apply that framework to homeopathic remedies. In 1988 the agency issued guidelines stating that "homeopathic drugs cannot be offered without prescription for such serious conditions as cancer, AIDS, or any other requiring diagnosis and treatment by a licensed practitioner. Nonprescription homeopathics may be sold only for self-limiting conditions recognizable by consumers. . . . [Their] labeling must adequately instruct consumers in the product's safe use." But what can safe use mean, if a product doesn't work?

It is the opinion of CU that the FDA should require homeopathic products to meet the same standards required of other drugs.

On the Fringe

Several fad diagnoses and treatments are out of step with current medical knowledge. Typically, their proponents use invalid diagnostic tests and charge high fees. Instead of attempting to prove their ideas to the scientific community, they have been marketing them directly to the public through books, magazine articles, talk-show appearances, and lectures. At the same time, they often attempt to alienate people from scientific health care by minimizing its benefits and exaggerating its risks.

"Orthomolecular Therapy"

Orthomolecular medicine is defined by its proponents as "the treatment of disease by varying the concentrations of substances normally present in the human body." It is said to have begun during the early 1950s when a few psychiatrists began adding massive doses of nutrients to their treatment of severe mental problems. The original substance used was vitamin B_3 (nicotinic acid or nicotinamide), and the therapy was termed "megavitamin therapy." Later the treatment regimen was expanded to include other vitamins, minerals, hormones, and diets, any of which may be combined with conventional drug therapy and electroshock treatments. In 1968 chemist and Nobel laureate Linus Pauling coined the term orthomolecular, based on the Greek word *orthos*, which means "straight" (or "correct"). A CU consultant estimates that this approach has been adopted by a few hundred physicians and is being used to treat a wide variety of conditions, both mental and physical.

During the early 1970s a special task force of the American Psychiatric Association noted in a report that orthomolecular psychiatrists were using unconventional methods not only in treatment but also in diagnosis. The report's conclusion may be the most strongly worded statement ever published by a scientific review body:

> This review and critique has carefully examined the literature produced by megavitamin proponents and by those who have attempted to replicate their basic and clinical work. It concludes in this regard that the credibility of the megavitamin proponents is low. Their credibility is further diminished by a consistent refusal over the past decade to perform con-

trolled experiments and to report their new results in a scientifically acceptable fashion. Under these circumstances this Task Force considers the massive publicity which they promulgate via radio, the lay press and popular books, using catch phrases which are really misnomers like "megavitamin therapy" and "orthomolecular treatment," to be deplorable.

The Research Advisory Committee of the National Institute of Mental Health reviewed pertinent scientific data through 1979 and agreed that megavitamin therapy is ineffective against mental problems and may be harmful. No comprehensive review of orthomolecular therapy for other conditions is known of at CU, and it is held in low regard throughout the scientific community.

"Hypoglycemia"

Some afflictions, such as arthritis and cancer, are so widespread and distressing that their victims are natural targets for ingenious promoters of quack cures. Working the other side of the street are those who exploit people with a variety of general symptoms by fitting them all neatly into a single diagnostic category. Over the years, "hypoglycemia"—low blood sugar—has been a favorite diagnosis of the medical fringe. This real but uncommon condition is often attended by symptoms of shakiness, trembling, tension, fast heartbeat, headache, sensations of hunger, weakness, and mental confusion. But in the vast majority of cases diagnosed as hypoglycemia by fringe practitioners, these symptoms are bodily reactions to anxiety, not hypoglycemia.

The overdiagnosis of hypoglycemia got much of its impetus

from the teachings of John Tintera, M.D., a physician who practiced about 30 years ago in Yonkers, New York, and Carlton Fredericks, a food faddist who wrote several books and hosted a popular radio talk show in New York City. Dr. Tintera's involvement with hypoglycemia followed publication in 1951 of *Body, Mind and Sugar,* by E. M. Abrahamson, M.D., and A. W. Pezet. The book, which has sold hundreds of thousands of copies, blamed low blood sugar for chronic fatigue, allergies, asthma, rheumatoid arthritis, neuroses, alcoholism, and suicide, as well as "the moral breakdown that underlies all delinquency and crime." The authors conceded that their views were not accepted by the medical profession but said that this was "largely because most doctors have not yet had time to read the literature."

In a series of medical journal articles published during the late 1950s and early 1960s, Dr. Tintera went beyond Dr. Abrahamson's claims and recommended periodic (and costly) injections of adrenal cortical extract ("ACE")—a relatively weak extract of hog and beef adrenal glands—for hypoglycemia. Dr. Tintera and his followers claimed that low blood sugar was caused by "tired" or "worn out" adrenal glands, and that ACE injections would remedy the problem.

ACE had been used as a treatment for Addison's disease, a serious disorder involving atrophy of the adrenal glands, but its use was already obsolete, having been supplanted by the isolation and synthesis of cortisone in the early 1950s, by the time it was first touted for hypoglycemia. In the 1970s it was evident that ACE was not effective for any disease.

Carlton Fredericks claimed that at least 20 million Americans suffered from hypoglycemia. Robert Atkins, M.D., author of *Dr. Atkins' Diet Revolution* and *Dr. Atkins' Health Revolution,* says that the majority of Americans experience it. But the American Diabetes Association states that the condition is uncommon except for reactions from injected insulin or oral drugs used to treat diabetes.

Some practitioners who diagnose "hypoglycemia" in large numbers of patients don't even bother to test them, whereas others misinterpret test results. The standard glucose tolerance test involves ingestion of 50 to 100 grams of glucose followed by repeated measurements of blood glucose levels. Endocrinologist Lynn J. Bennion, M.D., author of *Hypoglycemia: Fact or Fad*, calls the test "a six-hour bleeding session . . . where white-clad leeches sweeten the experience with an initial bottle of glucose syrup." Ingestion of so much sugar is an abnormal situation unrelated to the circumstances of most patients' symptoms. During this unnatural stress, notes Dr. Bennion, up to 25 percent of normal individuals (especially women) will develop low blood sugar. Moreover, test results can vary widely when the test is done repeatedly. The only way to reliably diagnose hypoglycemia is to prove that blood sugar is abnormally low when symptoms occur during the patient's usual living pattern. The most practical way to do this is probably with a home testing device. If hypoglycemia is documented, a cause must be sought. The evaluation should be guided by an endocrinologist.

"Candidiasis Hypersensitivity"

Candida albicans (sometimes referred to as monilia) is a normally harmless yeast found in the mouth, intestinal tract, and vagina. Under certain conditions, it can multiply as a so-called yeast infection on the surface of the skin or mucous membranes, but these infections are usually minor. Promoters of "candidiasis hypersensitivity," including some physicians, claim that even when infection is absent, the yeast can trigger multiple symptoms—and the list is long: fatigue, irritability, constipation, diarrhea, abdominal bloating, mood swings, depression, anxiety, dizziness, unexpected weight gain, difficulty in concentrating, muscle and joint pain, cravings for sugar or alcoholic beverages, psoriasis, hives, respiratory and ear problems, menstrual problems, infertility, impotence, bladder infections, and prostatitis.

According to its promoters, candidiasis hypersensitivity afflicts 30 percent of Americans. It is also being touted as an important factor in AIDS, arthritis, multiple sclerosis, and schizophrenia as well as hypoglycemia, and "mercury-amalgam toxicity." Some practitioners who espouse the concept of "candidiasis hypersensitivity" diagnose it in all or most of their patients.

The main promoters of "candidiasis hypersensitivity" have been C. Orian Truss, M.D., of Birmingham, Alabama, author/publisher of *The Missing Diagnosis*, and William G. Crook, M.D., of Jackson, Tennessee, who wrote and published *The Yeast Connection: A Medical Breakthrough*. According to Dr. Crook, "If a careful check-up doesn't reveal the cause for your symptoms, and your medical history [as described in his book] is typical, it's possible or even probable that your health problems are yeast-connected." He also claims that tests such as cultures don't help much in diagnosis because "Candida germs live in every person's body. . . . Therefore the diagnosis is suspected from the patient's history and confirmed by his response to treatment."

Dr. Crook claims that the problem arises because "antibiotics kill 'friendly germs' while they're killing enemies, and when friendly germs are knocked out, yeast germs multiply. Diets rich in carbohydrates and yeasts, birth control pills, cortisone and other drugs also stimulate yeast growth." Many of these facts are scientifically true. Nevertheless, it does not follow that an increase in yeast growth weakens the immune system. To correct these alleged problems, he recommends allergenic extracts, antifungal drugs, vitamin and mineral supplements, and diets that avoid refined carbohydrates, processed food, and (initially) fruits and milk.

Dr. Crook's book contains a 70-item questionnaire and score sheet to determine how likely it is that health problems are yeast-connected. Shorter versions of this questionnaire have appeared in magazine articles and in ads for products sold through health food stores.

The American Academy of Allergy and Immunology, which is the nation's largest professional organization of allergists, has issued position statements strongly criticizing the concept of "candidiasis hypersensitivity syndrome" and the diagnostic and treatment approaches used by its proponents. In addition to finding the concept of yeast allergy to be "speculative and unproven" (a polite way of saying it's rubbish), the allergists conclude: (1) its basic elements would apply to almost all sick patients at some time or other because its supposed list of symptom indicators is large; (2) overuse of oral antifungal agents could lead to the development of resistant germs that could pose problems; (3) adverse effects of oral antifungal agents are not uncommon and require periodic testing; and (4) neither patients nor doctors can determine the effectiveness of a treatment method without controlled trials. (Dr. Crook has said that he is too busy to test his theories.)

Owing largely to Dr. Crook's promotion, public interest in "candidiasis hypersensitivity" has grown rapidly. Several other books on the subject have been published. Some health food sellers now offer food supplements that are "yeast-free" and thus presumably "safer" than ordinary ones. Manufacturers, including several that market exclusively through chiropractors, are offering such products as *Candi-Care, Candida*

Cleanse, Candida-Guard, Candistat, Cantrol, Yeast Fighters, Yeast Guard, Yeastop, and *Yeast-Trol.*

In 1989 the FDA seized a supply of *Cantrol* from its manufacturer (Nature's Way Products, Springville, Utah) and issued a Health Fraud Bulletin instructing its field offices to initiate action against other illegally marketed "anti-Candida" products. Early in 1990 the FTC announced that Nature's Way had signed a consent agreement to stop making unsubstantiated claims that Cantrol is helpful in controlling yeast infections caused by *Candida albicans.* The FTC had charged that a 14-question "Yeast Test" promoted by the company could not determine that a person is likely to have a yeast infection and that there was no reasonable basis for claiming that Cantrol was effective against yeast problems. The agreement also required Nature's Way to pay $30,000 to the National Institutes of Health to support research on yeast infections.

These federal actions should deflate the market for bogus "anti-Candida" products. But the "candidiasis hypersensitivity" fad is likely to continue unless and until state licensing boards take vigorous action against the practitioners who are fostering it.

Chelation Therapy

Chelation therapy involves intravenous administration of a synthetic amino acid called EDTA into the bloodstream. EDTA is legitimately used to treat cases of heavy metal poisoning, including lead. According to its enthusiasts, EDTA supposedly cleans out unwanted minerals from various parts of the body before exiting through the kidneys. A course of treatment consisting of 20 to 30 injections can cost thousands of dollars. Chelation therapy is used most often in cases of heart disease, but its promoters also claim it is effective against kidney disease, arthritis, Parkinson's disease, emphysema, multiple sclerosis, gangrene, psoriasis, and other serious diseases. However, no controlled trials have shown chelation to be of help with any of these conditions. In 1985 the American Health Association concluded that chelation therapy is unproven for heart disease and can be dangerous as well.

A controlled trial whose protocol was approved by the FDA is now underway to test whether chelation therapy is effective against intermittent claudication, a condition in which impaired circulation to the legs causes pain when the person walks. Critics of chelation therapy believe that no benefit will be found.

Bogus "Nutritionists"

According to information gathered by CU consultants, during the past decade several unaccredited correspondence schools and other organizations have issued thousands of "degrees" and certificates. Holders of these credentials typically represent themselves as "nutrition consultants" and work in health food stores, chiropractic offices, or in independent practice, where they suggest dietary changes plus costly supplementation with vitamins, minerals, herbs, enzymes, glandular extracts, and the like. Many of them use hair analysis to diagnose "mineral imbalances," computerized questionnaires to diagnose "nutrient deficiencies" and other invalid tests to diagnose "food allergies." They are also prone to make inappropriate diagnoses of hypoglycemia, "candidiasis hypersensitivity" and chronic fatigue syndrome. Since nutrition is so much in vogue today, their activities may seem credible to some laypersons.

To combat this problem, dietitians throughout the United States have been spearheading legislation to achieve licensure for themselves and to restrict the practice of nutrition and use of the word *nutritionist* to qualified practitioners. So far, about half the states have passed laws regulating the practice of nutrition.

Some of the practices described in this chapter have great potential for harm. Consumers are advised to stay away from anyone who espouses any of them.

4

The Vitamin Pushers

Surveys suggest that nearly half the people in the United States pop a vitamin pill either regularly or occasionally—and some take a handful every day. Annual sales of vitamins in this country are close to $3 billion a year.

The vitamin marketplace is crowded. Hundreds of companies are selling thousands of "dietary supplements" through pharmacies, health food stores, supermarkets, department stores, person-to-person sales, and through the mails. Vitamins are sold individually and in a multitude of combinations that may include minerals, amino acids, and other substances.

Most vitamin users, concerned that their diet may not be adequate, take their daily doses as "insurance" against deficiency. Others—operating on the mistaken theory that if some is good, more must be better—hope that the products will provide extra energy, prevent disease, protect against stress, or enhance athletic ability.

What Vitamins Are—and Aren't

A vitamin is an organic (meaning carbon-containing) substance required to promote one or more essential biochemical changes within living cells. Unlike foods, vitamins are needed only in very minute amounts, and they do not provide energy (calories). For a substance to qualify as a vitamin, its absence must cause a specific deficiency disease that is cured when the substance is replaced. (Lack of vitamin C, for example, causes scurvy.) It may take weeks or months for signs of deficiency to show up.

There are thirteen known vitamins required by humans. Nine are water-soluble (C and the eight "B-complex" vitamins—thiamin, riboflavin, niacin, folic acid, B_6, B_{12}, biotin, and pantothenic acid), and four are fat-soluble (A, D, E, and K). Do any more vitamins remain to be discovered? Probably not, since patients on intravenous feeding fortified with only these vitamins have survived for years. Hucksters have touted "vitamin P" (bioflavonoids), "vitamin B_{15}" (pangamic acid) and "vitamin B_{17}" (Laetrile), but they are not true vitamins.

How Much Does a Person Need?

The Food and Nutrition Board of the National Academy of Sciences' National Research Council (NAS/NRC) publishes guidelines known as the Recommended Dietary Allowances (RDAs). These are defined as the levels of intake of essential nutrients "considered adequate to meet the known nutrient need of practically all healthy persons." The most recent RDA values were issued in October 1989.

The RDAs are recommendations—not "minimums" or "requirements." The level for each nutrient is deliberately set higher than most people need. The RDA for each vitamin is usually derived by estimating the range of normal human needs, selecting the number at the high end of that range, and adding a safety factor. The values vary somewhat by age and sex and are increased for women during pregnancy and while breast-feeding.

For two vitamins—biotin and pantothenic acid—the latest RDA report lists "estimated safe and adequate intakes" rather than RDAs. This was done because part of people's need for these vitamins is supplied by bacteria within the intestines; how much must come from food is not known.

The FDA took the Food and Nutrition Board's 1968 figures and simplified them to create the U.S. Recommended Daily Allowances (U.S. RDAs). These are the figures that appear on the labels of vitamin bottles and many processed foods. U.S. RDAs generally represent the highest level of the NRC's Recommended Dietary Allowance for each nutrient. Therefore, few if any people need more than the U.S. RDA. Most people can do just fine on less. In July 1990, the FDA announced a proposal to replace the U.S. RDAs with a new system of "Reference Daily Intakes (RDI)" based on the 1989 RDAs. These amounts will still be more than most people need.

Why More Isn't Better

As noted, some vitamin users assume that if small amounts are beneficial, taking large amounts will do even more for them. But a brief look at how vitamins work should dispel this notion.

A water-soluble vitamin functions in the body as a coenzyme. When it reaches the cells that need it, it combines with a special protein called an apoenzyme to form the enzyme required to carry out certain metabolic functions. Without the vitamin, this metabolism would not take place. A cell can make only so much apoenzyme per day, and this amount usually is satisfied with the vitamin provided by a typical daily diet. Thus, ingesting more of a water-soluble vitamin that has no apoenzyme to combine with cannot serve a vitamin function.

Fat-soluble vitamins help regulate specific metabolic activity. Like water-soluble vitamins, excess amounts of fat-soluble vitamins have no vitamin function to perform.

Although excess amounts of vitamins don't function as vitamins, they can still exert chemical (drug) effects. Whereas small amounts of excess water-soluble vitamins are usually excreted in the urine without problems, large doses can be harmful. Unlike water-soluble vitamins, excess fat-soluble vitamins are not easily excreted and tend to accumulate in the liver and in fatty tissue. Large doses, particularly of A and D, can do serious damage. Prolonged excessive intake of vitamin A can cause headache, pressure on the brain, bone pain, and damage to the liver. Excess vitamin D can cause kidney stones. Under medical supervision, however, certain vitamins can be useful as drugs in a few clinical situations.

Some vitamin advocates suggest that everyone should take dietary supplements to be sure of getting enough. They say, for example, that "eating on the run" and "overprocessing" of foods place the typical American in danger of deficiency. Some also cite "soil depletion" and dieting as reasons for needing vitamin supplements.

Medical consultants for CU believe that such claims are without merit. It's true that eating on the run, skipping entire meals, and watching one's weight have become common for many Americans. But it's unlikely that those habits are breeding vitamin deficiencies.

Take fast foods, for starters. In June 1988, when *Consumer Reports* last looked at McDonald's, Burger King, Wendy's, and their cohorts, it observed that "by choosing with an eye to damage control," fast-food meals can be fairly well balanced, especially if people use the salad bar, go easy on dressings and other fat-laden condiments, and choose milk (especially the nonfat variety) instead of a shake. The main problem with fast food is not what's missing but what's there—a lot of calories, sodium, and fat.

Skipping meals? Certainly many people do. But people who eat only one or two meals daily during the week usually more than make up for any deficits with snacks and with increased variety and abundance on weekends.

Dieting should be done sensibly, of course. But only prolonged or highly unbalanced diets could create risk of vitamin deficiency, CU's medical consultants say.

The argument about "overprocessing" of foods oversimplifies a complex issue. Processing can remove some vitamins and other nutrients. But it can also restore them or add new ones. B-vitamins lost during the milling of flour, for example, are restored by fortification.

Consultants for CU scoff at the idea that depleted soil robs the American diet of vitamins. Whereas a plant's mineral content may be influenced by soil composition, its vitamin content is largely determined by the plant's heredity. A carrot grown in depleted soil may be physically stunted, but its vitamin A content per unit weight will be the same as if it had grown in enriched soil.

Finally, some vitamins are lost in cooking. But losses of that sort are usually only partial and can be compensated for by including uncooked fruits and vegetables in the diet.

"Nutrition Insurance"

The suggestion to buy "nutrition insurance" in pill form can be very appealing. In 1985 a flyer from General Nutrition Corporation, which operates more than 1,000 health food stores, stated the case simply: "It would take a computer and a good deal of conscious effort to devise a diet that each day would give all the nutrients in optimum amounts. . . . From the viewpoint of . . . nutrition, a complete supplement may be the best possible buy in health insurance."

But experts disagree. "Vitamin pushers use deception by omission," states Victor Herbert, M.D., professor of medicine at Mount Sinai School of Medicine in New York City and a member of the NAS/NRC RDA committee from 1980 to 1985. "They list all the terrible things that can happen if your diet is lacking. But they never tell you that vitamin deficiency is rare unless a person's diet is extremely unbalanced. Most important, they never tell how to measure whether or not your diet is adequate. If they did, they'd lose customers. Determining dietary adequacy is actually quite easy."

Easy and undramatic. People can get adequate amounts of all essential nutrients by planning meals to include what nutritionists call the Basic Four Food Groups. The *average* daily intake should include:

• Four servings of vegetables, fruits, and fruit juices, at least one of which should be fresh.
• Four servings of grain and cereal products (including cereals, breads, rice, macaroni, and the like).
• Two to four servings of meats, fish, poultry, eggs, or beans.
• Two to four servings of milk or dairy products.

Because foods within each group differ in nutrient content, choosing a variety within each group is important. Adhering to the recommended minimum, with reasonable portion sizes, would provide about 1,200 calories and adequate amounts of all essential nutrients. Since most people eat more than that, it should be clear that eating a wide variety of foods from the Basic Four will easily provide the required nutrients. Further, though some advocates would lead people to believe otherwise, a few days without one nutrient or another will do no real harm. Supplements may be appropriate for pregnant or nursing women, children under two, strict vegetarians, and people with certain illnesses. But the decision to use supplements is best made with the advice of a doctor.

The "Vitamin Gap"

In 1989 the Council for Responsible Nutrition (CRN), which represents major manufacturers and distributors of dietary supplement products, began suggesting that virtually everyone has a "vitamin gap." Through ads in 20 magazines, it invited readers to take a seven-question "National Vitamin Gap Test." The ads stated that a negative answer to any of the questions may indicate a gap for various vitamins, minerals, or fiber—and that "vitamins fill the gap." But none of the questions were valid indicators of vitamin shortage. (One question, for example, was "Do you eat two servings of fruit per day?" Fruits are a rich source of vitamins A and C, but so are many vegetables. So someone eating fewer than two daily portions of fruit might still get adequate amounts of these vitamins from other foods.) Moreover, even if a shortage should exist, the problem is best remedied by dietary improvement, not by supplements.

More recently, Great Earth Vitamin Stores, the nation's second largest health food store chain, began inviting people to complete a 29-question "Nutrition Fitness Profile" and have it analyzed by a "highly trained vitamitician" at one of its stores. That way, said the company, "you can be confident that your special requirements are satisfied with a nutritional regimen featuring fully guaranteed vitamins and supplements of unsurpassed quality." A few of the 29 questions involve important health considerations (e.g., smoking, drinking, exercise, and blood cholesterol level), but none of the questions provide any basis for vitamin supplementation.

Hype About Stress

Another ploy in selling vitamins has been to offer protection against "stress." While some vitamin promoters refer only to physical stresses, others include mental stress, overwork, and the like. And some make no health claims at all but rely on the word *stress* in the product's name to sell it. Typical "stress-formula" vitamin products contain 10 or more times the RDA for vitamin C and several of the B-vitamins. These amounts probably are not high enough to cause trouble, but neither will they benefit anyone already getting near-RDA amounts from food.

After surveying the stress-formula marketplace in 1985, *Consumer Reports* noted the following claims in ads or product literature:

• Sears Shop at Home Service, which marketed Puritan's Pride stress formulas, asserted that "active lives subject us to considerable stress. Working hard and even playing hard create one type of stess. The weather even affects us. Colds and illness make more demands on our bodies. Of course the everyday pressures of life bring on emotional stress. All these types of stress increase your body's need for vitamins."

• The I. Magnin department store chain recommended *Clientele Stress Control Nutrients* "if you're very active, deal frequently with decision-making or just find yourself drained from everyday events."

• A flyer from General Nutrition Corporation included "traffic jams, arguments, meeting fast-approaching deadlines, or simply trying to decide what to wear at a party" as sources of stress that "can take their toll on various nutrients in our body, especially vitamin C and B-complex vitamins."

• Hoffmann-La Roche, which wholesales most of the vitamin ingredients used in vitamin preparations compounded by other manufacturers, advertised that "if you drink, smoke, diet or happen to be sick, you may be robbing your body of vitamins."

• Ayerst Laboratories, stating that "just being alive is stressful," suggested *Beminal Stress Plus* to avoid "stress burnout," a vitamin-deficiency state to which "nobody is immune."

• Lederle Laboratories—makers of *Stresstabs*—warned for years that "stress can deplete your body's store of water-soluble vitamins" and that "daily replacement is necessary."

According to Lederle, the market leader, the concept of high-dosage stress vitamins is based on a 1952 NAS/NRC report that recommended extra vitamins for people suffering from stresses such as general surgery, serious burns, and major fractures. However, that report explicitly stated that "in minor illnesses or injury where the expected duration of the disease is less than 10 days and when the patient is essentially ambulatory and is eating his diet . . . a good diet will supply the recommended dietary allowances of all nutrients."

Nutrition experts advise that although vitamin needs may rise with certain physical conditions, they seldom rise above the RDAs—and are easily met by eating a proper diet. Someone who is under enough stress to incur vitamin deficiency would probably be sick enough to be in a hospital. But ads for stress vitamins generally have been aimed at well-nourished members of the general public.

No evidence exists that emotional stress increases the body's need for vitamins. Lederle's chief of nutritional science stated emphatically that his company did not recommend *Stresstabs* for psychological stress. "We make it clear in our ads that we're talking about physical stress," he told a CU reporter. He also told the reporter that "people who eat a balanced diet do not need stress vitamins—or for that matter, any vitamin supplement at all."

To be sure, ads for *Stresstabs* made no mention of emotional stress. But they did picture an executive working at a paper-strewn desk after dark and touted the product "for people who burn the candle at both ends"—a phrase that some people might interpret as suggesting emotional as well as physical stress.

In 1986, after action by the New York State attorney general, Lederle paid $25,000 to the state and agreed not to make unsupportable claims that emotional stress causes depletion of water-soluble vitamins, that *Stresstabs* will reduce the effects of psychological stress, or that consumers undergoing ordinary physical stress cannot obtain all necessary nutrients by eating a well-balanced diet or taking an ordinary potency (meaning about 100 percent of the U.S. RDAs) multiple vitamin supplement.

The New York attorney general also persuaded E. R. Squibb & Sons to pay $15,000 in costs and to modify the claims made on the packaging of its *Theragran Stress Formula*. Squibb had been claiming that the product helps relieve stress resulting from "the complications of everyday life" and that "taking the recommended daily allowance [will] reduce the effects of psychological stress." Its ads had also suggested that biotin—one of the components of *Theragran Stress Formula*—is difficult to obtain in an average diet. In fact, biotin deficiency is virtually nonexistent. Except in infants, biotin deficiency has been reported only in individuals who ate unbalanced diets containing large amounts of raw eggs, which contain a substance that blocks biotin absorption.

Ask the Pharmacist?

In 1985 the FDA and the Pharmaceutical Advertising Council began a major campaign of public-service ads attacking quackery and encouraging people to ask their doctor or pharmacist about claims that seem too good to be true.

Curious about what advice pharmacists give their customers about vitamins, in 1985 CU sent reporters to 30 pharmacies in Pennsylvania, Missouri, and California. Posing as potential customers, the reporters complained either of feeling tired or of feeling tense or nervous. They asked a pharmacist in each store if a vitamin product might help. Vitamins are not appropriate treatment for stress or tiredness, and they should have been told as much. But 17 of the 30 pharmacists recommended vitamins as a solution for either stress or tiredness, one recommended L-tryptophan, an amino acid (see page 54), and only nine mentioned the possibility of seeing a physician. One recommended *Stresstabs* for fatigue because "that's what they have for when you burn the candle at both ends" while another said that a tired individual eating a balanced diet should take a supplement anyway because that person "might not be absorbing the food."

To explore how pharmacists are taught to handle such inquiries, CU sent questionnaires to the deans of all 72 pharmacy schools in the United States. All but one of the 51 who responded said this situation is covered in such courses as pharmacy practice. Almost all thought that pharmacists should attempt through questioning to identify possible causes of tiredness or nervousness and should ask whether a physician had been consulted. More than half said that pharmacists should advise that vitamins are unlikely to help either condition.

Hype for Athletes

Athletes, from the bodybuilding professional to the weekend jogger, may be tempted to pop vitamin pills to achieve better performance or to replenish vitamins lost through vigorous activity.

A cascade of advertising hypes vitamins for athletes. *All American Sports Vitamins* have been said to contain vitamins and other substances "to help you get the absolute maximum out of every ounce of sweat, every hour of training." Twinsport's *Endurance* products—endorsed by Robert Haas, author of *Eat to Win*—have been claimed to help realize your potential "whether you're a world-class athlete or a weekend recreationalist." Solgar has said its *Joggers* tablets are formulated "to give an edge to the serious competitor and endurance athlete." And Ayerst has suggested that even a two-mile jog is reason to replenish vitamins and minerals with *Beminal Stress Plus*.

It is true that strenuous exercise increases the need for calories, water, and a few nutrients. However, vitamin needs are unlikely to rise above the RDA amounts available from a balanced diet. The notion that extra vitamins are useful to athletes is also tied to the idea that extra vitamins provide extra energy—which is untrue. Energy comes from the calories in food, and vitamins have no caloric value.

A few companies—even more fanciful—have marketed vitamin supplements supposedly formulated for specific sports or fitness goals. The latest of these are "ergogenic aids," combinations of various vitamins, minerals, amino acids, and other substances claimed to enhance athletic performance. More than 100 companies are marketing them.

Ads for such products typically display men with huge muscles, and many contain endorsements from bodybuilding or weight-lifting champions. Perhaps the most brazen promotional campaign has been for Schiff's "Ergogenic Pro-Formance System"—a product line that includes *Formula 420 Daily Base* ("unsurpassed bodybuilding and energizing fuels"), *Formula 560 Ergogenic Energizer* ("antistress, energizing formula to help the body increase endurance"), and *Formula 300 Daily Annex* ("to give the extra . . . edge for ultimate endurance and performance").

Schiff began promoting these products during 1988 with colorful full-page ads in health food industry trade publications announcing that "The Biggest Names in Fitness Join Forces. The National Academy of Sports Medicine [NASM] and Schiff Sports Nutrition create the most advanced fitness program on earth." The ads and product brochures listed "a Blue-Ribbon NASM Board" of five prominent professionals in sports medicine, including Donald Cooper, M.D., a member of the President's Council on Physical Fitness.

Curious about this, CU obtained a copy of NASM's incorporation papers and contacted its "board" members for comment. Our investigation revealed that the "academy" was not a medical organization but a private corporation chartered in October 1988 for "research, education, new product development, exploration and explanation of new technology [and] consulting." All five "board" members said that although they had agreed to be listed in NASM literature, they had neither endorsed the advertised products nor given Schiff permission to use their names in any way. In fact, said Dr. Cooper, "I think the products are of no real value. A well balanced diet can supply all the nutrients and energy that an athlete needs. The only way to reach your maximum potential as an athlete is through hard work and practice. There are no safe shortcuts or miracles in capsules or tablets."

Hype for Smokers

Smokers are known to have lower blood levels of vitamin C than do nonsmokers, which has led some promoters to suggest that smokers should take extra vitamin C. But according to Dr. Herbert, "There is no credible evidence that smokers need more than RDA amounts of vitamin C. The 1980 RDA amount (60 mg) was at least four times as much as a normal person would ever need in a day."

In 1989 the RDA for vitamin C for smokers was raised from 60 milligrams per day to 100 milligrams per day—an amount still readily obtainable from a balanced diet. But according to Dr. Herbert, the change was "a political decision not backed by scientific evidence."

Moreover, Alfred E. Harper, Ph.D., professor of biochemistry and nutrition sciences at the University of Wisconsin, who chaired the NAS/NRC's RDA Committee in 1974, has pointed out that "most subjects used in the major experiments that served as the basis for present vitamin C allowances were smokers, [and so] the suggestion that smokers need high doses of vitamin C seems incongruous. If anything, it would seem much more appropriate to suggest that nonsmokers need less."

Hype for Seniors

In October 1986 *Consumer Reports* took issue with the American Association of Retired Persons (AARP), which operates the largest nonprofit mail-service pharmacy in the world (its gross sales are over $200 million per year). To promote *Activitamins*, AARP Pharmacy Service catalog had claimed that "a vigorous lifestyle puts extra demand on your body. So if you play golf or tennis or swim, walk, jog or bike, you should know about our formula." Calling this claim "bunkum," CU also criticized AARP for selling bee pollen, royal jelly, bone meal, several amino acids, kelp, alfalfa, rutin, and biotin "despite lack of any scientific evidence that using such substances as supplements serves any nutritional need."

After discussions with the National Advertising Division of the Council of Better Business Bureaus, AARP said that it would stop publishing the misleading claims for *Activitamins*, but it continued to sell the product as well as other questionable items. In 1987 AARP Pharmacy Service appointed a professional advisory board to offer advice and consumer messages about vitamin, mineral, and supplement products. Following the board's appointment, products with potentially toxic doses of vitamin A were reformulated, misleading product claims were stopped, and some dubious products (including protein supplements) were withdrawn from the pharmacy service's catalog. But alfalfa, lecithin, bone meal, garlic oil capsules, and brewer's yeast continued to be sold. In the March 1990 catalog, the page listing them contained a disclaimer: "Considerable controversy exists among experts on the merits of the nutritionals listed on this page. We offer quality products such as these as a convenience to interested members." Translated freely, this appears to be saying: this stuff may not be worth much, but if we don't offer it to you, you might decide to waste your money buying it somewhere else. So we'll sell it to you, as a convenience.

The AARP Pharmacy Service catalogs state that "a number of our most popular vitamin and mineral supplements . . . were developed exclusively for AARP members. They are not like ordinary vitamins." Among the exclusive preparations: "VitamInsurance," "Megavitamin," "Activitamins," and four "Stress Formula" preparations. All of these contain amounts of some ingredients that exceed the RDA.

Present in AARP's 1989 catalogs but missing from the March 1990 catalog was L-tryptophan. This amino acid is notorious because some users were damaged a good deal more than just in their pocketbooks. The product had been promoted by the health food industry to treat sleeplessness, depression, premenstrual syndrome (PMS), and overweight, although it had not been proven safe and effective for these purposes. On the contrary: in 1989 it was implicated in an outbreak of eosinophilia-myalgia syndrome (EMS), a rare blood disorder characterized by severe muscle and joint pain, weakness, swelling of the arms and legs, fever, skin rash, and an increase in a certain type of blood cell (eosinophile) in the blood count. Several states banned the sale of L-tryptophan supplements, and the FDA asked manufacturers to withdraw them from the marketplace. By May 1990 more than 1,500 cases of EMS were reported, with 23 deaths. The FDA recalled all products containing more than 100 milligrams of L-tryptophan, calling its continued availability a major public health problem.

Genuine Nutritional Shortages

Although vitamin deficiencies are rare among people who eat a reasonably varied diet, a fair number of Americans may need more of certain minerals. Some people should pay special attention to the following three:

1. *Fluoride* intake throughout childhood helps build decay-resistant teeth. The most efficient, economical way to get it is through fluoridated water. Parents of children who grow up in nonfluoridated communities should ask their dentist or physician about supplementary fluoride.

2. *Calcium* deserves particular attention because inadequate calcium intake is a factor in the development of osteoporosis ("thinning" of the bones), especially in women. Those who like milk, cheese, and other dairy products may get what they need from diet alone. But those consuming little calcium-rich food should seek advice on supplementation from a physician or registered dietitian.

3. *Iron* is needed to make hemoglobin, the component in red blood cells that carries oxen to the tissues. Lack of sufficient iron can cause iron-deficiency anemia. Women who are pregnant or who menstruate heavily should be checked by a physician to determine whether they are anemic and if they should increase their iron intake or take iron-containing medication.

Vitamin Claims and Cautions

Some of the claims for various vitamins recall a wag's comment about second marriages—"a triumph of hope over experience."

• *Vitamin B$_{12}$ and feeling good:* Vitamin B$_{12}$ is essential for health, but it is readily obtained from foods of animal origin. Only people with disorders in which B$_{12}$ absorption is impaired and strict vegetarians who eat no milk, meat, cheese, or eggs may require B$_{12}$ supplementation. Even at high doses, B$_{12}$ is virtually nontoxic to humans. It has been falsely promoted for a host of complaints, including arthritic pain, dizziness, and loss of memory. Some physicians give patients B$_{12}$ injections—as placebos—to alleviate what the doctor feels are psychosomatic symptoms. CU's medical consultants take a dim view of that ruse, which lends a false aura of legitimacy to the practice and wastes the patient's money.

Nature's Bounty, a large seller of vitamin and nutritional supplements, is currently selling a vitamin B$_{12}$ gel, called *Ener-B,* that supposedly provides a burst of energy when you stick it up your nose. The company has claimed that the gel, which costs about a dollar per dose, delivers a B$_{12}$ boost not possible with tablets, adding, "You'll feel good about it, especially the morning after."

The FDA is dubious. Usually it considers vitamins to be foods and therefore not subject to the same rigorous testing and approval procedures as drugs. But whereas a food is something that is eaten, *Ener-B* is smeared inside the nose, and the vitamin is absorbed through nasal membranes directly into the bloodstream. Furthermore, product literature has made druglike claims for *Ener-B.* Flyers distributed to health food stores stated that it delivers up to 10 times the amount of B_{12} as regular supplements. Press releases warned of the dangers of pernicious anemia—"one of the few vitamin deficiencies that still kills Americans." In fact, pernicious anemia is not as common as the hype would have you believe. Those who are affected require monthly B_{12} injections and must be under a physician's care. Vitamin B_{12} deficiency develops slowly. Most healthy adults have a three- to five-year supply of B_{12} stored in their liver. But then most people don't buy B_{12} to treat anemia; they want that extra energy boost promised in the ads.

The FDA advised Nature's Bounty that *Ener-B* was a drug that was illegal to market without FDA approval. Nature's Bounty responded by petitioning the FDA to treat *Ener-B* as it does other supplements and classify it as a food. The FDA did not approve the petition, but the product is still being sold. As one FDA official told CU, "We know of no other food you stick up your nose." As of this writing, the case is still in litigation.

• *Vitamin C and colds:* Proponents—most notably Linus Pauling—have recommended taking vitamin C in daily dosages of 1,000 to 2,000 milligrams in times of health and considerably more at the onset of a cold. (The adult RDA is only 60 milligrams a day.) At least 16 double-blind studies have found no benefit from such vitamin C supplementation. The classic study was conducted by researchers at the University of Toronto. They divided 3,500 volunteers into eight groups. Two groups received 259 milligrams a day of vitamin C, two received 1,000 milligrams, and two received 2,000 milligrams. The final two groups received a placebo. The study concluded that vitamin C did not prevent colds at all but *might* help to *slightly* reduce the severity of cold symptoms. To achieve this mild benefit, a daily dose of 250 milligrams (about the amount in two eight-ounce glasses of orange juice) was enough. Higher doses provided no extra benefit.

Megadoses of vitamin C can be harmful. Too much vitamin C can produce diarrhea and diminish the ability of white blood cells to kill harmful bacteria. Megadoses may encourage the formation of urinary-tract stones. Urine tests for glucose can be thrown off, and the effect of anticoagulant therapy may be lessened.

Medical consultants for CU recommend that people who have been taking large doses of vitamin C and wish to stop should do so gradually. Infants born of mothers who took vitamin C during pregnancy may experience "rebound scurvy" owing to the rapid drop in blood levels of the vitamin after birth.

• *Vitamin C and cancer:* Dr. Pauling also believes that massive doses of vitamin C can prolong the life of cancer patients. This claim is based on a study he reported with Ewan Cameron, a Scottish physician. However, experts who analyzed the report concluded that the study was not properly designed. The study measured how long two groups of patients survived after being labeled "terminal." But the patients in the vitamin C group were not as sick as those in the control group at the time the designation was applied.

Researchers at the Mayo Clinic have conducted three clinical trials to test the effectiveness of vitamin C against cancer, each involving more than 50 patients in the advanced stage of the disease. Half the patients received vitamin C, half a placebo. The researchers found no differences in survival time, appetite, severity of pain, weight loss, or amount of nausea and vomiting.

• *Vitamin E and fibrocystic breast disease:* Several years ago, preliminary studies by a research team at Sinai Hospital of

Baltimore suggested that vitamin E supplements might help women with mammary dysplasia (also called benign fibrocystic disease of the breast). But two double-blind studies subsequently reported no significant benefit. In large doses, vitamin E can cause diarrhea, headaches, and muscle weakness.

• *Vitamin B_6 and breast disease:* This vitamin too is of no value for cysts or other benign breast lumps. Indeed, no vitamin supplement has ever been shown to be useful for this purpose. Taking high doses of B_6 can cause peripheral neuritis, a painful nerve disorder that may be irreversible (see below).

• *Vitamin B_6 for PMS:* High dosages of vitamin B_6 have been widely advocated as a treatment for premenstrual syndrome. The evidence supporting this practice is thin—mixed results in small-scale studies. Since water-soluble vitamins are *relatively* safe in large doses (compared with fat-soluble vitamins), some physicians have felt comfortable in recommending B_6 in the range of 200 to 800 milligrams daily. (The RDA for adult women is 1.6 milligrams per day.) During the past few years, however, medical journals have reported more than 100 cases of toxicity from B_6 supplementation, resulting in a condition called peripheral neuritis. The reported symptoms, some of which resembled those of multiple sclerosis, included numbness and tingling in the hands, difficulty in walking, and electric shocks shooting down the spine. Although all the afflicted individuals improved greatly when they stopped taking the vitamin, a few did not recover completely. Some had been taking less than 50 milligrams per day. Medical consultants at CU strongly advise against megadoses of vitamin B_6.

Many medications and techniques have been tried for PMS—ranging from megavitamins to biofeedback—but none has had much success. A possible reason is that more than

150 different symptoms have been associated with PMS. Despite a fair amount of clinical investigation, its cause remains unclear.

• *Niacin and cholesterol control:* Public attention has been focused on niacin by Robert E. Kowalski's book, *The 8-Week Cholesterol Cure*, published in 1987. The B-vitamin also known as nicotinic acid, niacin is relatively cheap. In high doses it is considered one of the safest cholesterol- and triglyceride-lowering drugs—*under medical supervision*. Troublesome side effects often occur, most commonly the "niacin flush"—intense reddening and itching of the face and upper body that usually diminishes after several weeks. High-dose niacin can also cause gastrointestinal upset, abnormal liver function tests, elevated blood-sugar levels, and, rarely, atrial fibrillation (rapid beating of the heart).

• *Vitamin B₁ and mosquitoes:* Several outdoor magazines have reportedly recommended ingesting vitamin B_1—thiamine—as an effective mosquito repellent. As CU reported, "it doesn't work. A mosquito will gladly take your blood with or without added vitamins."

Reported cases of vitamin toxicity are uncommon. But they are particularly ironic because most people who get into trouble with vitamins have essentially poisoned themselves in the pursuit of health.

Recommendations

Medical consultants for CU believe that the best way to get vitamins is from foods in a balanced diet. Vitamin supplementation may be appropriate for children up to two years old, for children who have poor eating habits, for some people on prolonged weight-reduction programs, for pregnant women, for strict vegetarians (those who avoid eggs and milk as well as meat), and for people with certain illnesses, as directed by a physician.

If the decision is made to take a daily multivitamin or multivitamin/mineral pill for insurance, select an inexpensive brand that costs no more than a few cents a day and contains no more than 100 percent of the RDA of any ingredient. (The percentage of the U.S. RDA is listed on the label.) For safety's sake, never take more than RDA amounts except on medical advice and avoid doctors or nutrition consultants who recommend vitamins as cure-alls.

Several things can be done to clean up the vitamin marketplace:

• The FTC and state attorneys general should clamp down on misleading advertising for "nutrition insurance," "stress tablets," "sports vitamins," and the like.

• The FDA should evaluate the claims made by promoters of these products and publicize its findings.

• The pharmaceutical industry should develop a code of ethics that includes voluntary standards for vitamin product formulations and advertising claims.

• Pharmacists, pharmacy educators, and their professional organizations should recognize the pushing of unneccessary supplements as an ethical issue that deserves their attention.

5

Foods, Drugs, or Frauds?

Many nutrition supplements are claimed—despite lack of scientific proof—to treat or prevent a variety of serious diseases, delay aging, boost immunity, or restore pep. You won't find these claims on most product labels. The treatment-and-prevention claims appear elsewhere: in pamphlets stacked nearby, in books available for browsing or purchase, or in "bag stuffers" given away at the checkout counter. The claims are also made orally to customers by health food store retailers and by distributors involved in person-to-person marketing.

For manufacturers and distributors of nutrition supplements with inflated claims, it makes good legal sense to keep the products separate from printed information about their claimed benefits. If a label merely says "take two tablets three times daily as a dietary supplement," the product may be legally marketable as a food or food supplement and not subject to the rules governing drugs. But a therapeutic claim—

"take two pills three times daily for relief of arthritis"—makes the product a "drug" subject to regulation by the FDA. A message needn't be on the label itself to be considered "labeling." When literature is used to convey information about the purposes of a product, any claims in the literature can be considered part of the product's label.

Under the law, any product "intended for use in the cure, mitigation, treatment or prevention of disease" is a drug. Drugs that are not generally recognized as safe and effective by experts are considered "new drugs" that cannot be legally marketed without FDA approval. If a product is marketed with illegal therapeutic claims, the manufacturer can be ordered to stop making the claims. The FDA can also initiate seizure of the product, obtain an injunction, and/or seek criminal penalties.

The amount of literature containing illegal claims varies considerably from manufacturer to manufacturer. Those wishing to minimize the risk of triggering regulatory action provide no printed information and assume that customers will be educated through other channels of communication. Other manufacturers distribute materials marked "for professional use" or "confidential," which retailers can use covertly to advise their customers. Less cautious companies distribute literature intended to be displayed or given to customers.

Many "dietary supplement" products bear a disclaimer saying that they are "not intended to replace the services of a physician." But the claims made for them, and the manner in which they are marketed, send an opposite message to buyers. Some "supplement" products can cause serious injury because they contain toxic ingredients or contaminants. Many others, though innocuous themselves, encourage the victims of serious diseases to medicate themselves with ineffective substances even when effective treatments exist.

The Health Food Store at CU

Many companies have been playing the drugs-as-foods game. To get a close look at how they do it, CU created its own health food store in 1984. The store operated in two different states under different names, to ensure all the products ordered were shipped in interstate commerce and thus subject to federal regulation.

Health food stores have a very convenient way of obtaining product information from manufacturers: trade publications contain reader service cards that enable retailers to request information from any advertiser simply by circling the numbers corresponding to the ads that interest them. The investigators at CU didn't use this method but made direct contact by mail or phone with more than 70 companies, including some that don't advertise in the trade publications. After surveying their catalogs and other product information, CU placed orders, along with requests for additional literature to help explain the products' uses.

In addition to more than 300 products, a great deal of literature was received during the five months CU ran its little store. Some of this literature contained astonishing medical claims. The products, of course, were not sold to consumers. Instead, they were evaluated by a seven-member panel of medical and legal experts. Examining one or two products from each company, the panelists judged whether each item was legally a drug; whether it was known to be effective for its claimed purpose; whether it posed a direct hazard to the user or an indirect hazard by encouraging users to abandon other forms of therapy.

The panelists' final judgment was whether the manufacturer or distributor was violating the Federal Food, Drug, and Cosmetic Act by marketing an illegal "new drug." The panel also judged whether the product was "misbranded" because its labeling (which included any accompanying literature) failed to provide adequate directions for its intended use or included misleading information. Misbranding and marketing a "new drug" are criminal offenses.

The panelists concluded unanimously that more than 42 companies were violating both major provisions of the Food, Drug, and Cosmetic Act. Five products were judged the worst of the entire bunch:

• *Liquid Citrus Bio-Flavonoid Complex*, which an accompanying flyer said could help people with: herpes sores, easy bruising or hemorrhaging, diabetic cataracts, capillary oozing during surgical procedures, abnormal clumping of red blood cells and blood platelets, cancer-producing processes, excessive inflammation, abnormal uterine bleeding, allergy symptoms in children, cystitis toxicity, capillary bleeding caused by anticoagulants, and menopausal symptoms.

• *Padma 28* tablets, which contained 22 herbs prepared "in accordance with the principles of Tibetan herbology" and were claimed to produce results in treating angina pectoris and peripheral arterial occlusion. In addition, the product was said to be effective for "disabilities of old age, especially in relation to reduced circulation, such as senility, poor memory, and depressed energy levels," and for "poor circulation in general, producing cold feet, numb or antsy feeling[s] in the arms and legs, stiffness of the joints." The panel considered *Padma 28* not only an indirect hazard but also a direct one because one of its ingredients was the poisonous herb aconite. This product is no longer on the market.

• *Meganephrine*, a "nutritional supplement" whose ingredients came mainly from animal innards. Each capsule contained "250 mg Adrenal; 40 mg Hypothalamus; 50 mg Pituitary; 100

mg Medulla concentrate; 250 mg Tyrosine (an amino acid)."
In the view of CU's medical consultants, these ingredients
would be no more helpful than a bite of a hamburger. But
the company's order form said *Meganephrine* was "especially
designed to offset adrenal insufficiency and also raise serum
noradrenaline levels." Does anyone really need a higher noradrenaline level? The CU consultants didn't think so. Noradrenaline is made not only in the adrenal glands but also in
nerve endings throughout the body. Deficiencies have not
been described in the medical literature.

• *DMSO (dimethyl sulfoxide)*, an industrial solvent that the
FDA has approved only for the treatment of interstitial cystitis,
an uncommon bladder disease. DMSO has not been shown
to alter the course of any other disease, and it is illegal to
market it for any other medical use. Nevertheless, proponents
claim it can provide miraculous relief from arthritis, cancer,
mental illness, stroke, multiple sclerosis, varicose veins, and
other ailments. Despite public education efforts by the FDA,
many people still obtain DMSO from nonmedical sources and
attempt to use it for treatment purposes.

A brochure put out by one company claimed that DMSO
was "one of the most effective anticancer agents known," that
it "has the properties desired in any cancer drug," and that
it has been "used successfully" with chemotherapy. The
brochure did contain one fact—that DMSO is capable of passing through body tissues, taking other products with it. But,
said CU's expert panel, that fact makes DMSO a direct hazard
as well as an indirect one. The brochure said that DMSO
could be administered orally (in orange juice) or rectally, in a
retention enema. According to CU's panel, rectal use could
be fatal. The "other products" DMSO can take with it could
include bacterial toxins carried through the intestinal wall and

into the bloodstream. For someone already weakened by cancer, the effect of the absorbed toxins could be life threatening.

The product instruction sheet also advised diabetics using insulin to "decrease the insulin intake by 40–50% during the DMSO treatment" and to consume sugar "regularly with the DMSO doses." For some diabetics, following this advice could produce acidosis, possibly progressing to coma.

• *Rheumoid,* identified as a "nutritional substance" containing seven herbs, an amino acid (L-cysteine), and potassium, was described as "a safe and effective alternative to the arthritis drugs currently in use." The manufacturer's catalog and product guide listed 292 diseases and conditions, ranging from Alzheimer's disease and angina pectoris to seizures, stroke, and warts—each supposedly treatable with "nutritional substances" marketed by the company. The biggest customers appeared to be chiropractors. Laws prevent them from writing prescriptions for FDA-approved drugs, but companies like this one offer them the chance to "prescribe" something. Chiropractic journals CU reviewed were full of ads for unapproved remedies.

"Glandulars"

Long a staple of quack health spas and clinics, "raw gland concentrates" are marketed through health food stores as well. As explained by one manufacturer's pamphlet, "The theory is that like cells help like cells." So swallowing capsules of raw adrenal concentrate, for example, will supposedly "bolster the function" of your own adrenal glands. "Raw glandulars" were marketed by several companies, generally without any therapeutic claims. So the panel considered the products to be legally marketed (though expensive) foods. But, at the panel's suggestion, CU sent out 13 of them for laboratory analysis and got back some interesting results: seven had unacceptable levels of bacterial contamination. It's immaterial whether such products are legally considered foods or drugs. Those with high bacterial content were adulterated and potentially hazardous.

More Violations

Among the more than 40 companies judged to be violating federal law was Michael Schwartz's company, then called Michael's Health Stuff, of McAllen, Texas. His contribution to better health: a salve claimed to eliminate viruses and treat warts.

You can call Michael Schwartz many things, but he's not a quitter. Three years after CU called attention to his company, the FDA ordered him to stop making illegal claims for various nostrums, including *Artho Tabs* (arrests arthritis), *Diab Tabs* (treats diabetes), and *Manpower Caps* (cures impotence).

In 1989 Texas Department of Health officials charged the company, now operating in San Antonio as Michael's Health Products, with making illegal claims for 37 such "dietary supplements." Within weeks, Schwartz agreed to a permanent injunction against making therapeutic claims without FDA approval. He also agreed to pay $15,000 in fines and costs.

Schwartz is one of seven founders of the Dietary Supplement Coalition, a health food industry group formed in 1989 to counter certain FDA enforcement actions. The coalition wants greater freedom to market supplement products as "foods." Its brochure states that it will not try to protect products marketed with therapeutic claims. But at least five of its founding firms, including Michael's, have made such claims.

Dubious Distributors

Thousands of Americans have become distributors for multilevel marketing organizations selling nutrition supplements. Distributors are eligible to buy products wholesale and sell them retail to neighbors, friends, and relatives. But to make big money, a distributor must sign up others as distributors—and help them get people to work, in turn, for them—to get a percentage of all sales made "downline."

It's easy to become a distributor of nutrition supplements. Just visit any of the "health expos" held regularly in major cities around the country. A reporter from CU attended expos in Philadelphia and New York and found dozens of booths filled with people explaining how to improve health and make good money at the same time. During 1984 and 1985 the reporter became a distributor for 11 nutrition-supplement businesses, including Nutrition for Life, Blue-Green Manna, and Herbalife. The vignettes that follow are based on his experience during several months as a nutrition-supplement insider.

Nutrition for Life

Nancy (not her real name), a distributor for Nutrition for Life, lived in a stately old Manhattan building. She ushered the fledgling distributor into her apartment on the sixteenth floor and showed him into the living room. Lining one wall were four shelves filled with pill bottles and boxes.

The products looked innocuous, with names like *Herbal Blend 8* and *Pau D'Arco Taheebo Tea*, until she explained what they're used for. *"Herbal Blend 8,"* she said as she plucked a bottle off the shelf, "cures diabetes." She said she knew of cases in which diabetics taking *Herbal Blend 8* have been able to come off insulin. The company can't make claims like that on the label, she said, "or the FDA would get after us."

The *Pau D'Arco Taheebo Tea* tablets, Nancy said, were for preventing or treating cancer. Taheebo, she said, "works with the immune system" and for that reason can also cure AIDS. She said she knew three patients who'd been on the taheebo and "every one has gotten over AIDS."

"Can I actually tell people that?" the novice asked.

"Theoretically, you shouldn't make medical claims," Nancy replied. "But I said it right off. It'll cure AIDS. Because it's true. Face to face, you can say anything you want." Emphasize testimonials, Nancy advised. Recite cases in which the products have conquered disease. The new distributor's own experience with a product will also help convince people, she said. "You can say that it helped you if it did. Or even if it didn't."

Nancy explained how easy it is to sell the Nutrition for Life product line. "Everyone knows someone who has cancer or heart disease," she said. "Find out the names of those people, call them up, and tell them about the products."

Blue-Green Manna

In the mid-1980s Victor Kollman was marketing blue-green algae for the treatment of allergies, herpes virus, arthritis, leprosy, Mediterranean fever, Alzheimer's disease, the general aging process, narcolepsy, sickle cell anemia, anorexia nervosa, and many other health problems. Not just any blue-green algae, but the species found in Upper Klamath Lake in Oregon. There it was harvested by K. C. Laboratories, freeze-dried, and sold to the world as *Blue-Green Manna*. Kollman owned K. C. Laboratories and was the discoverer of *Blue-*

Green Manna. About 25 items made up the Manna product line.

Eating algae is nothing new. Fish have done it for years. It formed a staple of the Aztecs' diet and is still eaten by lake-dwellers on the West Coast of Africa. But convincing people to eat algae for serious diseases takes a certain genius. Few miracle cures have ever cost so little to package and sold for so much. A "Starter Pack"—120 capsules of *Blue-Green Manna* and one ounce of *Mannacol* (an alcohol extract)—costs $53. The cost of the ingredients, as estimated by CU, was well under a dollar.

How does Manna work? The way Kollman explained it, the algae contain "neuropeptides." When swallowed, these neuropeptides both detoxify the body and provide "food for the brain." Experts consulted by CU knew of no factual basis for these claims.

Kollman boasted that his manna was free of impurities such as "bacteria, fungi, yeast or mold of any type." But a 1983 FDA lab analysis of five ounces of *Blue-Green Manna* found 15 whole or equivalent adult flies, 164 adult fly fragments, 41 whole or equivalent maggots, 59 maggot fragments, one ant, five ant fragments, one adult cicada, one cicada pupa, 763 insect fragments, nine ticks, four mites, 1,000 ostracods, two rat or mouse hairs, four bird feathers, six bird-feather barbules, and 10,500 water fleas.

In 1983 the FDA seized six *Blue-Green Manna* products as unsafe food additives. In resisting the seizure, Kollman swore under oath that he was an algae expert with a Ph.D. in biochemistry from Utah State University. The government took a deposition from the Utah State registrar, who said the university had no record of Kollman's Ph.D. In 1986, after numerous court skirmishes, a federal court judge issued a permanent injunction ordering Kollman and his associates to stop manufacturing, distributing, and selling blue-green algae from Klamath Lake, Oregon. During the trial leading to the injunction, Kollman claimed that his products were foods rather than drugs, but the judge concluded that "the cost of the . . . products, which exceeds $300 per pound, is so high as compared to other sources of the same nutrients that it is apparent that these products are not and are not intended to be used as a food."

Herbalife

Herbalife's products were marketed primarily for weight loss, but company literature suggested the herbs they contained were effective against a wide range of serious illnesses as well. When CU investigated, four of its basic products contained laxative ingredients. The amounts in the products might not produce trouble for everyone, but in 1985 an Herbalife spokesman told a U.S. Senate subcommittee that more than 40 percent of 428 surveyed users had reported "transient side effects," including 48 (11.3 percent) with diarrhea.

A few months before the Senate hearing, the California attorney general filed a consumer-protection lawsuit against Los Angeles–based Herbalife and four of its executives, including company president Mark Hughes. The suit accused them of "numerous unfair and illegal statements and practices," including making unapproved drug claims for some products, misrepresenting that the products' herbs will curb the appetite, and using a marketing plan that was an illegal pyramid scheme. In 1986, to settle the case, Hughes and the company agreed to pay $850,000 to the State of California and were ordered by the court to change their marketing plan, to limit testimonials, and to stop making a long list of unreasonable claims for their products.

Kurt Donsbach's Activities

One of the leading proponents of nutritional supplements for preventing and treating disease is Kurt W. Donsbach, whose activities have spanned virtually every aspect of selling, prescribing, promoting, publicizing, and lobbying for such products.

In 1970, while Donsbach operated a health food store, he was visited by undercover agents for the California health department. He variously prescribed vitamins, minerals, herbs, and cabbage tablets for breast cancer, spastic colon, serious heart ailments, and emphysema. He pleaded guilty in 1971 to one count of practicing medicine without a license and was fined $2,750.

In 1973 Donsbach was charged with nine more counts of illegal activity including misbranding of drugs and manufacturing drugs without a license. He pleaded "no contest" to one of the new drug charges and paid a $100 fine. As a condition of his probation, Donsbach agreed not to involve himself in the sales, manufacturing, or repacking of any drugs. In 1974 he was found guilty of violating his probation and was fined $200 plus court costs. From 1975 to 1989 Donsbach was chairman of the Board of Governors of the National Health Federation, a group described in Chapter 13 that lobbies aggressively for the health food industry. He has written more than 40 publications on nutrition, including 20 "Dr. Donsbach Tells You What You Always Wanted to Know About . . ." booklets, which he says have sold more than nine million copies. And, at various times, he has published newsletters, magazines, and journals, intended for the public and for various professionals (mostly chiropractors) who see things his way.

Donsbach founded and was president of Donsbach University, an unaccredited school that offered bachelor's, master's, and Ph.D. "degrees" in nutrition through correspondence courses. Donsbach himself sports a "Ph.D." degree from Union University, which is also unaccredited, in addition to his degree from an unaccredited chiropractic school. He also claimed to have graduated from the "Hollywood College School of Naturopathy" and had obtained a license to practice naturopathy based on what appeared to be a diploma. However, in 1990, education officials in Oregon concluded that his "diploma" was counterfeit because no such school had existed.

At the time CU investigated, Donsbach was also board chairman of Health Resources Group, which operated Nutrition Motivation (a multilevel company), HRG Distributors (which sold supplements through health food stores), Health Radio Network (which broadcast Donsbach programs via satellite hookup), and Health Resource Centers (two clinics in southern California). Products bearing Donsbach's name— sold through HRG and Nutrition for Life—included *Orachel* (an "oral chelation" product claimed to be effective against heart disease), *Prosta-Pak* (claimed to relieve prostate problems), and *C-Thru* (suggested for preventing cataracts).

One of Donsbach's inventions was the Nutrient Deficiency Test, a computer program used by some practitioners. Patients answer a 284-item questionnaire (e.g., "Do you catch cold easily?" "Is your tongue shiny?"). The program supplies a printout that diagnoses "nutritional deficiencies" and lists the supplements (obtainable from the practitioner) needed to correct them. An FDA chemist analyzed the test by feeding it questionnaires completed for perfectly healthy people of different ages and sexes. In all cases the printout said, "It appears that you have several nutrient deficiencies . . ." and recommended a long list of vitamins and minerals. Nutrition experts judged the test worthless.

Many of the "Dr. Donsbach Tells You What You Always Wanted to Know About . . ." booklets recommend massive doses of vitamins for diseases. In 1984 Donsbach was sued by Jacob Stake, of Urbana, Illinois, who charged that he had become ill and been hospitalized as a result of ingesting large amounts of vitamin A over a period of two and a half years. The suit papers state that Stake began taking the vitamin at age 16 because Donsbach's booklet on acne had recommended it. The case was settled out-of-court for about $35,000.

Currently Donsbach is operating a Mexican hospital that "specializes in the treatment of chronic, degenerative diseases including cancer and multiple sclerosis." He is also board chairman of the Confederation of Health Organizations, a group formed in May 1989 "to unite the major elements of the alternative holistic health movement."

Stronger FDA Action Is Needed

When a health product is marketed with illegal claims, the FDA can issue a regulatory letter specifying the law violations and demanding to know how the problem will be corrected. If the letter is ignored, or if the FDA decides to begin with more forceful action, the agency can initiate court proceedings for a seizure, injunction, or criminal prosecution. But civil actions don't effectively deter, because many manufacturers view dealing with them as merely part of the cost of doing business.

Criminal prosecution could have a strong deterrent effect because the guilty parties would be risking imprisonment in addition to these costs. But, as of this writing, the FDA had undertaken only two criminal prosecutions involving fraudulent nutrition supplements during the previous 25 years. Obviously, the agency hasn't done enough to deter food supplement quackery. It has defended this relative inactivity by pointing to its many other responsibilities and limited budget. But knowledgeable critics believe that criminal prosecution would be far more cost-effective than civil action.

It isn't often that a magazine does an undercover investigation and publishes the names of more than 40 companies that are committing crimes. But the May 1985 issue of *Consumer Reports*, in which CU reported on its "health food store" activities, did exactly that—in effect challenging the FDA to stop the violations.

Within days after CU's article was published, the FDA distributed a "Talk Paper" stating that "many of the products mentioned in the article were known to the FDA and were under investigation, covered by the OTC drug review, or already acted upon by the agency. Those new to the agency will be scheduled for coverage in the future." But it turned out that only four of the companies named by CU were under investigation, 10 had been subjected to FDA enforcement action, and 25 were "not known" by the agency to be involved in illegal activities. Further analysis of this information revealed that the proceeding against one company "acted upon" had taken place 23 years previously and that several others had continued to break the law despite what the agency had done. Moreover, information about eight of the 25 "unknown" companies had been mailed by an outside investigator to the FDA's Health Fraud Branch as well as to its commissioner and chief enforcement officer months before CU's article was published.

The investigation by CU had collected evidence regarding hundreds of products being marketed with illegal therapeutic claims. The FDA never asked for this evidence and stopped only a few of the violations that CU revealed.

Since 1985 FDA activity against health frauds has increased somewhat. The agency has cosponsored two national health fraud conferences and more than 20 regional ones. In addition, it has distributed information packets to thousands of newspapers, magazines, and radio and television stations, urging them to reject fraudulent ads. However, it has not brought any new criminal cases against companies marketing "food supplements" with illegal therapeutic claims.

Unless the FDA adopts a *deterrent* approach by prosecuting criminal offenders, the problems described in this chapter will continue to flourish.

6

Allergies:
Real or Bogus?

The ad in *Respiratory Times*, a physicians' trade journal, featured a solitary, empty chair in a doctor's waiting room. The doctor, according to the headline, was suffering from "patient deficiency syndrome." But relief for this financial malady was at hand. The ad, for a California laboratory, urged doctors to "cure" the problem by treating their share "of America's 35 million Allergy Sufferers."

A CU reporter who saw the ad in 1987 decided to investigate. He found that a number of such laboratories had opened in recent years and that all work the same way. The doctor mails in a sample of a patient's blood. The lab analyzes it to identify the patient's allergies and then sends a printout of the results to the doctor, who may order extracts to use in allergy shots. In this way, doctors with little or no training in allergy can boost their income by treating allergic patients with shots instead of recommending drugs or referring the patients to allergy specialists.

Just how well do these labs diagnose allergies? To find out, the reporter asked a CU medical consultant to draw some blood from him and send it to three testing laboratories—in New York, Arizona, and California. Then he asked two New York City allergists to test him for allergies.

Both allergists found him allergic to dust, ragweed, trees, grasses, and mold. In the case of mold, one said it was a slight allergy, the other said it was moderately severe. Those results were no surprise. The reporter customarily experienced mild allergy symptoms for a few weeks each spring and fall; he either ignored the sneezes and sniffles, knowing they'd be short-lived, or took an over-the-counter antihistamine.

The allergists who tested the reporter detected no signs of any allergic reactions to food, and the reporter had never experienced any. But two of the three mail-order labs identified food allergies as well as the reporter's grass allergy. (None picked up his allergies to dust, ragweed, trees, and mold.) One lab reported a "strong food allergy" to cow's milk and the "suggestion of food allergy" to beef. The other reported allergies to beef, eggs, cod, and salmon—a surprise, since fish is the reporter's favorite food.

An erroneous mail-order diagnosis can lead to costly and potentially hazardous treatment—a series of injections that set the patient back several hundred dollars a year for two or more years. Such shots are unnecessary for most hay-fever victims, and they don't work against food allergies. But mail-order diagnosis is only one of the pitfalls facing unsuspecting allergy sufferers. Abuses range from the overuse of skin tests and allergy shots to the treatment of nonexistent food allergies. Those individuals who have allergies, as an estimated 20 percent of Americans do, should be wary before turning themselves over to a shot doctor.

The Profit in Shots

Many experts agree that shots have a place in allergy treatment, but only for carefully selected patients. Too often, they say, shots are overused, and many people who get them don't need them. One reason is that shots are more profitable than other allergy treatments. Patients treated with shots may need to see the doctor every week or month for several years, whereas those on drugs come to the office only once or twice a year.

A former president of the American Academy of Allergy and Immunology told CU that only 20 to 25 percent of his allergic patients had symptoms severe enough to justify shots. "The rest can be controlled very nicely with drugs," he said.

Allergy experts say that far too many patients are put on shots simply because they have positive skin or blood tests. Often these people don't have allergy symptoms, say the experts. Moreover, overzealous skin-testing increases anyone's chances of getting a falsely positive result. Indeed, some doctors go overboard on skin tests, sometimes performing 100 or more in a single visit—a practice that escalates their fees. The American Medical Association's Council on Scientific Affairs recently stated that the number of skin tests "should rarely exceed 50."

Even significant allergies may not warrant shots. For example, a skin test may suggest that a person is extremely sensitive to Bermuda grass. But this is a problem only if that person lives in the South or California, or visits there in the summer. If not, shots are unnecessary.

One of the major abuses involving allergy shots is treatment that goes on too long. A patient should expect to see improvement after one year, or two years at the most, say CU's medical consultants. Shots that aren't working should never continue beyond two years.

When shots do work, they should continue for three to five years, after which they usually can be stopped. About half the time, relief from symptoms will persist indefinitely. If symptoms recur, another course of shots can always be undertaken.

Immunity Gone Wrong

Allergy symptoms can range from merely annoying to life threatening. Most victims have hay fever or "allergic rhinitis." Less common problems include asthma, skin diseases such as atopic eczema, and food allergies.

Whatever the symptoms, the underlying cause is the same—a glitch in the body's immune defenses. The immune system protects against disease-causing germs, such as bacteria and viruses. But allergic people have an immune system that also reacts to harmless material, such as pollen, as if it were a threat.

The tendency to become sensitized to pollen or other allergens is largely inherited. Initial encounters with an allergen may prompt the body to form antibodies, which deploy on specialized cells called mast cells. When coated with antibodies, mast cells are like explosive mines bristling with detonators. Millions of them lie in the respiratory and digestive tracts and in the skin, waiting for the right allergen to come along. When one does, the mast cells explode, releasing powerful chemicals such as histamine. These engage the "invader" but can also inflame nearby tissues, provoke hive formation and narrowing of the airways, and stimulate mucus production in the nose and sinuses.

Usually, this translates into symptoms of hay fever, such as watery or itchy eyes, sneezing fits, and a runny or stopped-up nose. The main culprits here are pollens: primarily from trees in spring, grasses in early summer, and ragweed in late summer and early fall.

Many allergic people have mild hay fever that responds to self-treatment, primarily with antihistamines. Those drugs prevent histamine from exerting its noxious effects. Even nonprescription antihistamines, such as brompheniramine maleate, chlorpheniramine maleate, and pheniramine maleate, can relieve sneezing, itching eyes, and other symptoms. The drugs typically cause drowsiness, but taking them only before bedtime for the first few days may reduce that problem, and it may fade after a few weeks of use. Antihistamines are most effective if used before allergy symptoms become severe.

But antihistamines often don't work well against stuffy noses. So a hay-fever sufferer may also need a decongestant, which is taken by mouth or topically as nasal sprays or drops. Effective oral decongestants include pseudoephedrine and phenylpropanolamine. Many effective products for nasal use are available over the counter; they have to be used sparingly, though, because they can cause rebound congestion if applied more than two or three days in a row.

Some people need more than an over-the-counter remedy, however. They may suffer debilitating hay-fever symptoms for months or year-round. Or they may have asthma aggravated by allergies or even life-threatening reactions to certain insect stings. They require professional help.

Whatever the problem, the critical first step is a thorough medical history. The series of questions—what are the symptoms, when and where do they occur, and so on—may reveal that the problems actually arise from something other than an allergy.

If allergies are in fact present, the history can narrow the possibilities. Seasonal symptoms, for example, suggest that one or more pollens is at fault. Persistently recurring symptoms may point to some factor at home or work, such as mold, dust, or pets. A diagnostic test may also be needed to pin down the allergy more precisely.

The test most commonly used is a skin test, which detects antibodies the body has created against specific allergens. Typically, the doctor or an assistant uses a penlike instrument to make a series of pricks on the back or forearm. A drop of allergen extract is then placed on each puncture. Many different allergens can be tested in this manner. Alternatively, some specialists prefer to inject the extract directly into the skin.

A positive test produces a small, circular welt around the puncture or injection site within 10 to 20 minutes. The bigger the welt, the greater the sensitivity to the allergen. An alternative to skin testing is the blood test performed by mail-order labs. But a blood test is more expensive than skin tests and less sensitive or precise. Its only advantage is that it requires just a single puncture, making it more acceptable for some people.

Food Allergies Versus Food Intolerances

In a random sample of 3,300 American adults, 43 percent said they have some type of "adverse reaction" to foods, a reaction often ascribed to a food allergy. Pop-medicine publications have spread the word that food allergies are a major public-health problem, causing myriad physical and psychological symptoms.

Actually, food allergies are uncommon. Only about 5 percent of children and less than 2 percent of adults have true food allergies, in which a food provokes an immune response.

What people believe are food allergies are often food intolerances. Some of those are individual idiosyncrasies without a detectable physical basis: Uncle Gus's gas problem after eating Aunt Millie's corn muffins—but not someone else's. Millions of Americans report such food idiosyncrasies and get along simply by avoiding the offending food.

Some food intolerances arise from well-identified causes. Many people have trouble with milk, for example, because they're deficient in an enzyme needed to digest lactose (milk sugar). They may experience bloating, diarrhea, or other abdominal symptoms from milk, cheese, ice cream, and other dairy products.

The distinction between food intolerance and food allergy is important. People with a mild food intolerance may be able to eat moderate amounts of a problem food with little discomfort. But those with a severe food intolerance or any form of food allergy must avoid the offending food at all times.

When people mistakenly believe they have food allergies, the results can be unfortunate. Life may become less enjoyable because the diet is restricted needlessly, and sometimes nutritional deficiencies may arise. So it's important to find out whether a genuine allergy is present.

The main culprits in true food allergies are cow's milk, protein, egg whites, various kinds of nuts, and, especially, seafood. Allergic reactions to any of them might include one or a combination of several symptoms: nausea, vomiting, diarrhea, rashes, itching, difficulty breathing. On rare occasions, even fatal reactions can occur. (Patients with proven food allergies are commonly advised to carry a dose of epinephrine, a prescription drug, with them in case of a severe reaction.) There's no scientific evidence, however, that food allergies cause psychological or behavioral problems.

Proper Diagnosis and Treatment of a Food Allergy

Skin tests done with food extracts sometimes provide useful information about the way a patient reacts to food. A negative test means that the patient is highly unlikely to be allergic. A positive test means only that the patient *might be* allergic. Confirmation requires either a well-documented history of allergic reactions to a food or a controlled oral "challenge" with the suspect food under the supervision of a physician.

A reputable allergist will say that there is only one effective treatment for a food allergy: avoid the food. Shots, they will say, are totally useless as a therapy for food allergies.

Dubious Approaches

Some physicians approach food allergies from a different perspective. They base a diagnosis on a "provocation" test, in which the food extract is injected into the arm or put under the tongue. They contend that food allergies *can* be treated, often with extracts that patients administer themselves.

Many of these physicians are ear, nose, and throat specialists who refer to themselves as "otolaryngic allergists." According to a pamphlet distributed by the American Academy of Otolaryngic Allergy in 1987, the list of possible disorders that can be caused by food allergies is almost endless. "Even more startling," continues the pamphlet, "is the mounting evidence that foods and chemicals may cause severe difficulties in the nervous system and in the mind itself." Then the good news: "Fortunately, most cases of food allergy can be helped" through the use of "modern procedures."

A second group of unorthodox allergy practitioners includes physicians of various stripes who call themselves "clinical ecologists." They contend that foods and chemicals trigger numerous physical and psychological problems. Advocates of this belief consider their patients to be suffering from "environmental illness," "total allergy syndrome," or "twentieth-century disease," which they say can mimic almost any other illness.

The symptoms of this ubiquitous malady are said to include depression, irritability, mood swings, inability to concentrate or think clearly, poor memory, fatigue, drowsiness, diarrhea, constipation, sneezing, running or stuffy nose, wheezing, itching eyes and nose, skin rashes, headache, muscle and joint pain, urinary frequency, pounding heart, swelling of various parts of the body, insatiable appetite and obesity, and even schizophrenia. Proponents state that virtually any part of the body can have "elusive symptoms for which no organic cause can be found."

Clinical ecologists speculate that the immune system is like a barrel that continually fills with chemicals until it overflows, signaling the presence of disease. Some, however, also say that "immune system dysregulation" can be triggered by a single episode of infection, stress, or chemical exposure. Potential stressors include practically everything that modern humans encounter, such as urban air, diesel exhaust, tobacco smoke, fresh paint or tar, organic solvents and pesticides, certain plastics, newsprint, perfumes and colognes, medications, gas used for cooking and heating, building materials, permanent-press and synthetic fabrics, household cleaners, rubbing alcohol, felt-tip pens, cedar closets, and tap water.

To diagnose "ecologically related" disease, practitioners take a history that emphasizes dietary habits and exposure to environmental chemicals they consider harmful. A physical examination and standard laboratory tests may be performed, mainly to rule out other causes of disease. Standard allergy test results are usually normal.

Treatment requires avoidance of suspected substances and may involve changes in life-style that can range from minor to extensive. Generally, patients are instructed to modify their diet and to avoid such substances as scented shampoos, aftershave products, deodorants, cigarette smoke, automobile exhaust fumes, and clothing, furniture, and carpets that contain synthetic fibers. In severe cases, patients may spend several weeks in environmental control units designed to remove them from exposure to airborne pollutants and synthetic substances that might cause adverse reactions. After fasting for several days, the patients are given "organically grown" foods and gradually exposed to environmental substances to see which ones cause symptoms to recur.

"Ecologically ill" patients may think of themselves as immunological cripples in a hostile world of dangerous foods and chemicals and an uncaring medical community. In many cases, their life becomes centered on their illness. Some companies are catering to these beliefs by offering such products as "no-fungicide" paints, "organic" clothing, and even specially outfitted travel trailers.

In 1986 Abba I. Terr, M.D., an allergist affiliated with Stanford University Medical Center, reported on 50 patients who had been treated by clinical ecologists for an average of two years. Despite treatment, 26 patients reported no lessening of symptoms, 22 were clearly worse, and only two improved. Among the prescribed treatments: 14 of the patients had been advised to move their home to a rural area, and seven had been told to use a portable oxygen tank. In 1989 Dr. Terr reported on 90 patients, including 40 from his earlier report. More than one out of three had been diagnosed as suffering from "candidiasis hypersensitivity" (see page 33).

Provoke and Neutralize

Otolaryngic allergists and clinical ecologists often use similar techniques for diagnosing and treating food allergies. One of these is the "intracutaneous provocative food test," which is supposed to provoke—and thereby detect—food allergy. The doctor injects a liquid food extract (chocolate, for example) into the patient's arm, then watches for symptoms—drowsiness, fatigue, chills, or any discomfort the patient reports. If no symptoms appear within 10 minutes, progressively stronger concentrations of the extract are injected.

When symptoms do occur, a weaker solution of the extract is then injected to "neutralize" the reaction. If that doesn't work, the doctor injects stronger solutions until the purported neutralizing dose is found—usually during the same all-purpose visit. That neutralizing dose is then used for food-allergy treatment.

The dose is administered if the patient expects to confront the food—chocolate cake at a party, for example. If the patient can't resist, neutralizing injections supposedly protect against an allergic reaction.

The extract can also be placed under the tongue—the "sublingual" method. Patients usually receive a bottle containing the neutralizing dose of the food extract and are told to put three drops under the tongue right before or after confronting a food.

One thing these techniques have provoked is a lot of skepticism. Several controlled studies have now evaluated them for efficacy. All concluded that the techniques are ineffective for diagnosing or treating food allergies. The most recent such test was reported on August 16, 1990, in *The New England Journal of Medicine*. Eighteen patients who had been diagnosed as allergic by experienced clinical ecologists were given provocation and neutralization tests using a double-blind protocol developed by researchers at the University of California. No difference was found between the symptoms following food extract injections and those that followed injections of dilute salt water. The researchers suggested that clinical ecology is "based on placebo responses."

In 1983 the Health Care Financing Administration (HCFA) proposed to exclude intracutaneous and sublingual methods from coverage under Medicare. The HCFA said both of the methods lacked "scientific evidence of effectiveness."

The HCFA proposal prompted the otolaryngic allergists to do a clinical study of those methods—which they had been using uncritically since 1961. The results were published in 1988. Before publication, CU obtained a copy and asked two board-certified allergists conversant in allergy research to evaluate the study. Both identified serious flaws in its methodology.

The California Medical Association, the American Academy of Allergy and Immunology, and a committee of the Ontario Ministry of Health have also assessed provocative testing and neutralization therapy. They all judged the techniques to be unproven. The American Academy of Allergy and Immunology described the techniques as having "no plausible rationale or immunologic basis."

In 1983 an FDA advisory panel on allergenic extracts concluded that food extracts are unsafe and ineffective for treating food allergies. The FDA is expected to announce that it has accepted the panel's findings. When that happens, neutralization treatment will constitute an unapproved use of food extracts. Physicians can still use the extracts any way they want, because the FDA can't dictate medical practice. But unapproved use of a drug increases a physician's vulnerability in the event of a malpractice suit.

Avoidance or Drugs

The most effective way to treat an allergy is to avoid what causes it. When avoidance isn't possible, the next best solution is medication to relieve symptoms. In recent years, new prescription drugs with reduced side effects have enhanced allergy treatment significantly: a new breed of antihistamines that seldom causes drowsiness; a liquid nasal spray, which CU's medical consultants report is quite effective in treating symptoms of both asthma and hay fever, works particularly well in children, and is notable for its near-total lack of side effects; steroid nasal sprays, which are particularly effective against nasal congestion. Optimal treatment may require a combination of drugs. According to CU's medical consultants, such therapy can relieve symptoms in all but the most severe cases.

The Time for Shots

When drugs fall short, the patient may be a candidate for allergy shots. The shots are effective against some allergens that are inhaled, such as pollens that cause hay fever or aggravate asthma, and against allergies to insect stings. To repeat: shots are *not* effective against food allergies.

Treatment begins with shots once or twice a week. The first injection contains a very dilute dose of an allergen, so as not to provoke an allergic reaction. Each succeeding shot contains a higher concentration. The aim is to increase the concentration gradually to maintenance dose—the highest concentration that the patient can tolerate without an adverse reaction, such as generalized itching or hives. The process of reaching a maintenance dose commonly takes from four to six months. After that, the patient receives monthly injections of the maintenance dose, generally for at least two years.

Allergy shots can work well when used appropriately. But even in the right situation, say CU's consultants, shots have drawbacks that should make them the treatment of last resort.

First, they contain allergens, so there's always the danger of an allergic reaction. An allergist who gives shots walks a fine line: improvements are greatest at the highest maintenance dose, but that's also the dose most likely to cause allergic reactions. In very rare cases, such reactions can be fatal.

The hazards of allergy shots stem partly from the uncertain quality of their extracts. In contrast to other types of drugs, most allergenic extracts lack uniform standards of potency, and in some instances the differences are significant. For example, the dust extract sold by one company may be as much as a thousand times stronger or weaker than a similar extract sold by another. That could be dangerous, especially if the doctor were to switch from a weaker to a stronger extract in the course of treatment.

So far, only about a dozen of the 1,500 different extracts on the market have been standardized. They include some of the most important ones, however, such as short ragweed, several grasses, cat, and house-dust mites (the major allergen in house dust).

Even when successful, shots usually fail to provide complete relief; patients often need drug therapy as well.

Which Extracts Work?

• *Insect stings.* The best results with shots occur in people who experience serious reactions from insect stings. Studies show that allergy shots provide almost complete protection against harmful effects from subsequent stings.

• *Ragweed.* Most other immunotherapy research has looked at ragweed, the major cause of hay fever. Well-controlled studies show that shots for ragweed pollen work about 85 percent of the time. Shots are also effective against hay fever caused by grasses, mountain cedar, and dust mites. The efficacy of other extracts, though, ranges from probable to dubious.

In 1974 the FDA convened a panel of allergy experts to review the efficacy of such extracts. The panel concluded in 1985 that many of the 1,500 marketed extracts were effective for diagnostic use in skin tests. Their value in treatment, however, was far less certain. The panel found convincing proof of efficacy for only a handful. Nevertheless, because of the efficacy of ragweed extract, the panel concluded that extracts of other inhalant allergens would probably work also.

Here's the current status of some other commonly used extracts:

• *Pollens.* Although clinical studies are lacking for many pollens, such as birch, oak, red maple, annual bluegrass, and others, most authorities believe that these extracts are effective.

• *House dust.* Some allergy experts say these extracts work; others strongly disagree. The raw materials for several such extracts come from the contents of vacuum-cleaner bags. Analyses show that the extracts contain anything from dog and cat dander to allergens associated with dust mites, rodent hairs, molds, and other substances. Because of the lack of consistency from one batch to another, the FDA advisory panel concluded in 1986 that house-dust extracts are potentially unsafe and should be taken off the market. The FDA has not yet acted on the advisory panel's recommendation.

• *Mold.* A few studies that evaluated mold extracts produced inconclusive results. Allergy experts CU spoke with said they prefer to treat mold allergies with drugs whenever possible.

• *Cats.* An estimated 58 million cats live in 27 million American homes, and many people are sensitive to them. Until recently, researchers thought the problem was mainly cat dander. Now they know that most people allergic to cats are also sensitive to the saliva cats apply to themselves when grooming.

Three clinical studies—two in the United States, one in Scandinavia—show that shots allow people to tolerate cats for longer periods. Yet many of these people remain quite sensitive. Medical consultants for CU say that cat-extract shots may help people who are exposed to cats occasionally, perhaps when visiting friends who own one. But such shots are totally ineffective for allergic people who live with a cat. For those people, the most effective measure is to find another home for the cat. If that's not feasible, keeping the cat out of the bedroom may offer some relief.

Asthma and Allergies

Should asthmatics get allergy shots? Some doctors think so, but such treatment remains controversial. Many of America's 15 million asthmatics do have allergies—about half of the adults and 90 percent of children. Yet some people with the worst asthma have no allergies at all.

Avoidance is the best treatment when allergies provoke asthma. Pets and dust often cause problems; removing them may offer dramatic gains.

Today's drugs, the second line of defense, usually control the wheezing, coughing, and shortness of breath that occur in asthma. Bronchodilators, for example, make breathing easier by widening bronchial tubes that have been narrowed by muscle spasm, inflammation, and mucus. Asthmatics with mild asthma can often obtain short-term relief with over-the-counter bronchodilator sprays containing epinephrine. Longer-acting bronchodilator sprays that require a prescription include those containing albuterol or terbutaline. Theophylline, another long-acting bronchodilator, is taken orally or intravenously. Other prescription drugs that alleviate asthma include steroid and cromolyn sprays.

Some asthmatics—those not helped by avoidance or drugs and whose attacks are serious enough to require hospitalization—might be candidates for allergy shots. But their allergies must first be documented. Asthma can be triggered by many factors besides allergies, including exercise, stress, respiratory infections, cold weather, and cigarette smoke. Current evidence suggests that shots may be worth a try in carefully chosen patients, particularly those with allergies to dust mites, grasses, and cats.

What to Do

For those seeking help with allergies, CU advises visiting a board-certified allergist who does not espouse the dubious beliefs and practices described in this chapter. A suitable referral may be obtainable through your family physician. Credentials may be checked by calling the American Board of Allergy and Immunology in Philadelphia (215-349-9466) or consulting the *Directory of Medical Specialists* at a hospital or public library.

A Last Resort

Before resorting to shots, say CU's consultants, the doctor should first determine the following:

• The symptoms have lasted for at least two years—long enough to indicate a chronic rather than a temporary problem.
• The symptoms disrupt the patient's life. They're severe and persist for several weeks or months each year.
• Neither avoidance nor medication is effective.
• There is evidence that shots will work against the particular allergies.

Allergists do make exceptions. An opera singer, for example, may need shots to be entirely free of symptoms. An airline pilot may want shots in order to avoid any sedating effects from drugs.

For most patients, though, drugs are preferable. For one thing, they cost less. At an average of $20 per shot, a typical series of shots plus a consultation will come to about $400 a year. Drugs are usually needed for only a few weeks or months each year. Drugs also work faster. In hay fever, for example, antihistamines may produce results within a few minutes, chromolyn sprays take about two weeks, while shots usually take six months or more to build up an effective dosage.

7

Dubious Cancer Therapy

Each year, according to estimates made by the American Cancer Society, half a million Americans will die of cancer and close to one million new cases will be discovered. (Another half million will be diagnosed with superficial skin cancers not included in these figures because they are easily detected and cured.) The society also estimates that one out of four people presently living in the United States will eventually develop cancer but that half could be saved with early diagnosis and current treatment methods.

Although heart disease kills far more people, cancer is the most feared of all diseases. "In fact," says Ernest H. Rosenbaum, M.D., medical director of the San Francisco Regional Cancer Foundation, "some patients react to the diagnosis of cancer in much the same manner that people in primitive societies react to a witch doctor's curse—as a sentence to an inevitable and ghastly death." They fear that the treatment will be unpleasant, costly, and mutilating, that they will become disabled and helpless, and that they will be abandoned by other people.

Cancer quacks cater to these feelings by appearing optimistic and encouraging their patients to take an active role in their treatment. In addition, many of today's dubious cancer treatments seem consistent with both popular and scientific beliefs about diet, life-style, and the relationship of mind and body.

Active participation in treatment can help people feel more in control of their life whether or not the treatment is effective in the long run. However, any psychological lift from following a bogus method should be weighed against the loss of time and money involved, as well as the disillusionment that may occur later.

"Unproven" Versus Proven Cancer Treatments

What distinguishes proven (orthodox) from unproven (unorthodox) cancer treatment? To be considered proven, a treatment must be tested in enough biopsy-diagnosed cancer patients to demonstrate that those who receive it do better than those who don't. So far, no drug that has failed laboratory tests has ever been proven effective against human cancer. For this reason, human trials are normally not done unless tests in animals or tissue cultures yield favorable results. Promoters of dubious cancer treatments rarely collect any data that could show whether their methods are effective.

The term *cancer* describes more than 100 diseases characterized by abnormal cell growth. Each type of cancer has its own characteristics. Some tumors grow slowly and remain localized, whereas others grow rapidly and metastasize (spread to distant sites through the bloodstream or lymphatic channels). For these reasons, any method claimed to be effective against *all* cancers should be viewed with skepticism. Cancer researchers do not expect to find such a "magic bullet" in the foreseeable future.

Testimonials Can Mislead

People tend to believe what others tell them about personal experience. And many people who feel that an unorthodox method has helped them enjoy sharing their success stories with others.

Some people who give testimonials have simply been tricked. A striking example of this was presented at the quackery hearing conducted by Representative Claude Pepper in 1984. Carl Barnes, M.D., a pathologist from Florence, Alabama, described what happened after his father-in-law learned that he had incurable cancer of the lung. Troubled by severe bone pain due to the spread of the cancer, the man traveled to a clinic in the Bahamas for immuno-augmentative therapy— a series of injections that cost several thousand dollars. During his stay, his chest was X-rayed and he was informed that the tumor had become smaller. That his pain persisted was attributed to the therapy doing its work. He returned home "with a total euphoria," Dr. Barnes told the Pepper subcommittee, "and told everyone he was cured." Unfortunately, he was not. The clinic's X-ray film was overexposed, Barnes noted, which had made the tumor appear to be smaller. Reexamination at an Alabama hospital proved that the tumor had not shrunk, and death occurred two months later.

Immuno-augmentative therapy (also called immune augmentation therapy or IAT) was developed by Lawrence Burton, Ph.D., a zoologist who claims to treat cancer by manipulating protein components he says are part of the patient's immune system. Burton says he extracts these components from blood with a process he has patented. However, Saul Green, Ph.D., a former Memorial Sloan-Kettering Hospital biochemist who is renowned for his work in protein chemical analysis, states that it is not possible to isolate the substances Burton claims to use by the techniques described in the patents. In 1977, after failing to complete a satisfactory application to the FDA to test humans in the United States, Burton established a clinic on Grand Bahama Island. In 1980 he received an enormous boost when CBS-TV's "60 Minutes" suggested that a patient treated by Burton appeared to be making an amazing recovery. The patient died a few days after the program was shown, but "60 Minutes" never informed viewers of this fact.

Burton's treatment involves daily injections of serums prepared from the pooled blood of cancer patients or healthy donors. In 1985 public health officials found antibodies to the AIDS virus in vials of serum obtained from several patients—suggesting that blood infected with the AIDS virus had been used to prepare IAT treatment materials. Antibodies to hepatitis B (a serious liver infection) have also been found in IAT serum, and several cases of this disease have occurred following treatment at Burton's clinic.

What about individuals who undergo unorthodox treatment and live for years to tell about it? When cases of this type are investigated, it usually turns out that proven treatment also has been administered but is not getting the credit it deserves. For example, several cases have surfaced of people whose cancer had been confined to a polyp in their large intestine. This so-called Stage One cancer can usually be cured by inserting an instrument (sigmoidoscope) into the rectum and snipping or burning off the polyp. The patients who survived benefited from this traditional procedure but credited the unconventional treatment they had been undertaking at the same time. In addition, although statistics exist for "average survival times," the course of cancer in individual cases is often unpredictable. Thus, when patients who have used unorthodox therapy live longer than they or their doctors expect, a quack may get undeserved credit.

Dubious Methods

Dubious methods can be classified in eight broad categories: corrosive agents, plant products, special diets, drugs, correction of "imbalances," "vaccines," devices, and psychological approaches. Some promoters combine one another's techniques in a "shotgun" approach to make their wares more marketable. Here are some examples of these methods.

The Black Salve

In recent years, scientists have found chemicals that can destroy certain superficial skin cancers. Except for that, such corrosive agents are worthless and can result in serious burns. Nevertheless, salves, poultices, and plasters have been applied directly to tumors with the hope of burning them away.

Ruth Conrad, of Blackfoot, Idaho, learned that the hard way. In the mid-1980s, acting on the recommendations of several acquaintances, she consulted a naturopath about a pain in her left shoulder. When she also called attention to a sore on her nose, he felt it, said it was cancerous, and gave her a black salve. During the next few days, her nose was painful and red streaks ran down her cheeks. When she reported this to the naturopath, he replied that this proved she had cancer and to keep applying the salve. Within a week, a large part of her face, including her nose, sloughed off, and she required 17 operations over a three-year period to reconstruct her face. Subsequent investigation revealed that the naturopath was not licensed, that he had obtained the salve from a source in Mexico but did not know what was in it, and that there was no reason to believe that Ms. Conrad's sore was a cancer. The salve turned out to contain a corrosive chemical that ate away her skin like an oven cleaner. Despite all this, the naturopath maintained that if she had continued to follow his treatment for another week, her face would have healed normally.

Herbal Tea

Most folk remedies fall into the plant category. Many herbal teas are claimed to be effective when ingested or for bathing external cancers. ADS, described as an herbal tea, was sold for $125 to $150 per quart by Bruce Halstead, M.D., a California physician. Although Halstead maintained that ADS was a "nutritional supplement," analysis revealed it to be 99.4 percent water plus a brown sludge composed mainly of coliform bacteria (the type found in human feces). In 1986 Dr. Halstead was fined $10,000 and sentenced to four years in prison after being found guilty on 24 counts of cancer fraud and grand theft. Following his trial, the prosecuting attorney called him "a crook selling swamp water." At this writing, Dr. Halstead is appealing his conviction and remains free on $100,000 bail.

Pau d'arco, also known as ipe roxo or taheebo tea, is another popular cancer "cure" sold by mail and in health food stores as a "dietary supplement." It's also touted as a cure for AIDS. A daily teaspoonful of this tea supposedly will get rid of toenail fungus as well.

Dr. Varro Tyler, author of *The New Honest Herbal*, said this of pau d'arco: "Its lack of proven effectiveness, its potential toxicity, and its relatively high cost all render its use both unwise and extravagant."

The Gerson Diet

Many dietary approaches have been recommended for cancer, including fasting, megadoses of nutrients, consumption of raw foods, and various complicated dietary regimens. Proponents of the Gerson diet claim to accomplish "detoxification" by daily enemas and a diet consisting primarily of fresh fruit and vegetable juices. Salt, spices, sodium bicarbonate, alcohol, and tobacco are forbidden. After several weeks, milk proteins, vitamins, and various other food supplements are added. This program was developed by Dr. Max Gerson, a German-born physician who emigrated to the United States in 1936. It is still actively promoted by Gerson's daughter, Charlotte Gerson Straus, through lectures, talk show appearances, and publications of the Gerson Institute in Bonita, California. She claims that "by healing the body, you can heal cancer and almost any other chronic disease" and that "all chronic diseases are deficiency diseases." The treatment is available at a clinic in Tijuana, Mexico. Although its publicists claim high cure rates for various cancers, the clinic has not actually kept track of most of its patients.

Laetrile

Laetrile is one of several unproven remedies concocted by the late Ernst T. Krebs, Sr., a San Francisco physician. It is the trade name for the chemical amygdalin, a substance abundant in the pits of apricots and various other plants. Amygdalin is composed of two units of glucose, one unit of benzaldehyde, and one unit of cyanide. Laetrile is also referred to as "vitamin B_{17}," although it is not a vitamin. Physicians who treat cancer victims with Laetrile typically include it as a key component of "metabolic therapy."

Many animal studies have demonstrated that Laetrile has no beneficial effect against cancer. Between 1957 and 1975 the National Cancer Institute tested the substance on animal cancers on five different occasions. Four other independent cancer research centers also studied Laetrile and concluded that it is not effective.

Over the years, studies of case reports of humans have also been uniformly negative. In one done in the 1970s, Dr. Ernesto Contreras, a Mexican physician who had claimed to have treated more than 16,000 cancer patients with Laetrile, submitted 12 case reports to the FDA to illustrate his successes. Investigation by the FDA revealed that six had died of their disease, one still had cancer, and three could not be located. Two others had been treated with orthodox therapy, which made it impossible to tell whether Laetrile had helped them.

In response to political pressure, the National Cancer Institute in 1980 sponsored a clinical trial on patients with advanced cancer who had no hope of cure. The Mayo Clinic and three other U.S. cancer centers participated. Of 178 patients, not one was cured or even stabilized, and none had any lessening of any cancer-related symptoms. The median survival rate was 4.8 months from the start of therapy. In those still alive after seven months of treatment, tumor size had increased. Several patients experienced symptoms of cyanide toxicity or had blood levels of cyanide approaching the lethal range.

In 1975 a former cancer patient named Glenn Rutherford sued in federal court to stop the FDA from interfering with the sale and distribution of Laetrile. Although Rutherford's cancer had been confined to a polyp that was cauterized at a Mexican clinic, he told the court that Laetrile had cured him and was necessary for his continued survival. The district judge responded by issuing an injunction that permitted cancer patients to import a six-month supply of Laetrile for personal use if they could obtain a physician's affidavit that they were "terminal." (The affidavits were conveniently obtainable from companies that marketed Laetrile.) In 1979 the U.S. Supreme Court disagreed. The court reasoned that it is not possible to determine with certainty who is terminal, and that even if it were possible, both terminally ill patients and the general public deserve protection from fraudulent cures. In 1987, after further appeals were denied, the district judge finally yielded to the higher courts and terminated the affidavit system.

The Revici System

"Biologically guided chemotherapy," formerly called lipid therapy, is based on the notion that cancer is caused by an imbalance between constructive (anabolic) and destructive (catabolic) processes. Its main proponent has been Emanuel Revici, who was born in Rumania in 1896 and began practicing in New York City in 1947. Revici says he attended medical school in Rumania, but at this writing state licensing authorities are investigating whether he actually did so.

To treat the patient, Revici prescribes lipid alcohols, zinc, iron, and caffeine, which he says are "anabolic," and fatty acids, sulfur, selenium, and magnesium, which he classifies as "catabolic." His formulations are based on his interpretation of the specific gravity, pH (acidity), and surface tension of single samples of the patient's urine. Revici also claims success against AIDS.

Scientists who have offered to evaluate Revici's methods have never been able to reach an agreement with him on procedures to ensure a valid test. However, his method of

urinary interpretation is obviously not valid. The specific gravity of urine reflects the concentration of dissolved substances
and depends largely on the amount of fluid a person consumes.
The acidity depends mainly on diet but varies considerably
throughout the day. Thus, even when these values are useful
for a metabolic determination, information from a single urine
sample would be meaningless. The surface tension of urine
has no medically recognized diagnostic value.

In December 1983 Revici's license was suspended for 60
days while the New York Office of Professional Medical Conduct reviewed charges that he had promised cancer cures to
three patients. One was Edith Schneider, who had consulted
Revici after several other doctors had advised her to have a
marble-sized lump removed from her left breast. Revici persuaded her to undergo treatment with him. After 14 months,
the tumor had filled one breast and spread to the opposite
breast and to many lymph nodes—requiring removal of both
breasts and treatment with radiation and chemotherapy.

Ms. Schneider filed suit. Although a jury awarded her more
than a million dollars, the verdict was partially overturned by
a higher court. As a result, a jury will be asked to decide
whether she had assumed the risk of failure by undergoing
Revici's treatment instead of early surgery.

In 1988 another jury awarded more than $1.3 million to the
estate of another woman who suffered an agonizing death from
colon cancer under Revici's care. When she initially consulted
him, her tumor was the size of a marble and probably curable
by surgery. Evidence presented at the trial indicated that
although the tumor actually continued to enlarge, Revici said
it had gotten smaller and was almost gone. It was also revealed
that after the suit was filed, Revici allegedly doctored his
records to suggest that the woman's cancer was far advanced
when she first consulted him.

In response to the lawsuits and other complaints, state licensing authorities placed Revici on probation for five years. The terms of his probation bar him from treating patients for cancer unless they have been so diagnosed by another physician. Revici must then inform the patient that his treatment is unorthodox and urge the patient to consult a cancer specialist and a psychiatrist or psychologist before signing a consent form.

Harvey Wachsman, M.D., J.D., the attorney who represented both plaintiffs in the suits, believes that those probation terms do not protect desperate cancer patients. He urged that Revici's medical license be revoked immediately.

Livingston Vaccine

Vaccines have been prepared from various substances including pooled cancers, the patient's own blood and/or urine, animal blood and/or urine, and cultures of germs. A leading proponent of vaccine therapy is Virginia Livingston-Wheeler, M.D., who operates a clinic in San Diego, California. Her ten-day "Immu-Shield" program costs about $5,000. She postulates that cancer is caused by a bacterium she calls *Progenitor cryptocides*, which invades the body when resistance is lowered. To combat this, she claims to raise the body's resistance by administering vaccines prepared from cultures of the patient's urine or stool secretions plus standard bacterial vaccines. She also recommends eating a vegetarian diet, avoiding chicken, eggs, and sugar, taking various vitamin and mineral supplements, and "enhancing the immune response through visualization and stress reduction." Although she claims to have a very high recovery rate, she has published no clinical data to support this. Attempts by scientists to isolate the organism she postulates have not been successful. In February 1990, the California Department of Health ordered the Livingston-Wheeler Clinic in San Diego to stop treating cancer patients with a vaccine made from their own urine.

Simonton Method

O. Carl Simonton, M.D., who directs the Simonton Cancer Center in Pacific Palisades, California, claims that cancers may be affected by meditation. He suggests that the brain can stimulate endocrine glands to inspire the immune system to attack cancer cells. He and his associates have developed a system of relaxation and mental imagery that includes having patients imagine their cancer cells being destroyed by their own immune system. In 1988 the center's five-day program cost $2,800. There is no scientific evidence that visualization produces any physical benefit. Some observers have suggested that Simonton's program may have positive psychological effects because it may help people relax and give them a feeling that they are "doing something" positive. However, critics point out that false hopes can kill some people by deterring them from effective treatment and can prevent those who are incurable from making the best use of whatever time they have left.

Another person who preaches that emotions play a large role in the development of cancer is Bernie Siegel, M.D., author of *Love, Medicine and Miracles*. He suggests that disease can be cured if a depressed person can change an unhealthy perspective. But the prevailing scientific viewpoint disagrees. Researchers at the National Institute on Aging recently completed a 10-year study of depression and cancer in a random sample of more than 6,000 Americans. Those with depressive symptoms were found to have a cancer rate no higher than that of nondepressed people.

"Metabolic Therapy"

Harold Manner, Ph.D., a former biology professor who had left his academic position to market what he called "metabolic therapy," died in 1988. He had achieved notoriety in 1977 by claiming to have cured mice of cancer with injections of Laetrile, which was making headlines at that time. (What Manner actually did was digest the tumors by injecting them with a protein-dissolving enzyme along with the Laetrile—a technique that has no practical application to humans.) For the next decade, he promoted "metabolic therapy" for the treatment of cancer, arthritis, multiple sclerosis, and other serious diseases.

Dr. Manner defined metabolic therapy as "the use of natural food products and vitamins to prevent and treat disease by building a strong immune system." He theorized that chemicals in food, water, and air cause large numbers of primitive cells to become cancerous. When the immune system is functioning normally, the cancer cells are destroyed, he said. But if it is weakened by poor nutrition, environmental pollutants, or debilitating stress, they are uninhibited and multiply rapidly. Therefore, the way to treat cancer is by revitalizing the body's immune system with diet, supplementary nutrients, and "detoxification."

In 1982 Dr. Manner affiliated with a clinic in Tijuana, Mexico, which was later renamed the Manner Clinic. During 1988 the clinic charged $7,500 for its 21-day program of vegetable juices, "natural foods," intravenous Laetrile, coffee enemas, and large amounts of vitamins, minerals, enzymes, glandular extracts, and other concoctions.

Research by Barrie R. Cassileth, Ph.D., of the University of Pennsylvania Cancer Center, Philadelphia, indicates that "metabolic therapy" is a commonly used unorthodox cancer treatment. While its components vary from practitioner to practitioner, all base their approach on the idea that cancer and other chronic illnesses result from a disturbance of the body's ability to protect itself.

Although there may be a grain of truth to this idea, no one has ever been able to demonstrate that general immunity can be boosted by special diets, dietary supplements, or medications. Nor has any controlled study ever shown that "metabolic therapy" or any of its components has the slightest value in treating cancer or any other chronic disease. Although Dr. Manner claimed a 74 percent success rate in treating cancers, there is no evidence that he even bothered to keep track of how his patients did once they left his clinic.

Insurance Fraud

In 1988 a reporter on assignment for *Nutrition Forum* attended a Manner seminar for doctors (mostly chiropractors and naturopaths) and uncovered another seamy aspect of cancer quackery: insurance fraud. During the meeting, Ronald King, a claims supervisor for North American Health Insurance Coordinators, of Dallas, Texas, described how his company files insurance claims for "alternative health care" facilities in Mexico, the United States, Germany, and Greece.

Most insurance companies are reluctant to pay for unproven treatment. But King said that by using persistence and filling out claim forms with the "right" procedure codes, his company is able to collect on most of the claims it files. He indicated that instead of revealing the true nature of the treatment, his company sometimes substitutes a code number for a standard procedure. King said that North American keeps 16 percent of the amount it collects on behalf of its clients—one of which was the Manner Clinic. Manner added that his clinic was

billing insurers for this commission by calling it "administrative costs." Sure of the importance of his message, Manner
authorized the sale of tapes of the seminar to participants,
including the reporter.

Seek Help Through Reliable Channels

If a person has a question or needs medical attention for a
cancer or suspected cancer, the most prudent action is to seek
help through reliable channels. The family physician may be
a good starting point.

General information about cancer can be obtained from a
local chapter or the national office of the American Cancer
Society, as well as from the National Cancer Institute's Cancer
Information Service (CIS), Community Special Projects
Branch, Division of Cancer Control and Rehabilitation, 8300
Colesville Rd., Silver Spring, Maryland 20910. Another source
of information is the CIS Regional Cancer Centers, which can
be reached by calling 1-800-4-CANCER, except from Wash-
ington, D.C. (1-202-636-5700), Alaska (1-800-638-6070), or
Hawaii (1-800-524-6070).

Physicians can get up-to-date information about treatment
protocols and results—for both standard treatments and clinical trials—through the Physician Data Query (PDQ), a computerized database that is maintained and updated monthly
by the National Cancer Institute. This enables most doctors—
and hence their cancer patients as well—to benefit from the
latest scientific knowledge without having to travel far from
home.

8

The Mistreatment of Arthritis

The only well-preserved spine of a Neanderthal man is bent from arthritis. But when the first Neanderthal bones were discovered in 1856, arthritis treatment had advanced little beyond the caveman era. In the 1850s Americans with arthritis could choose among some 1,500 advertised "cure-alls," whose ingredients typically included flavored water, alcohol, narcotics, and/or various toxic substances. Today, although medical science has made great strides in many areas, there still is no cure for most forms of arthritis.

Because quackery thrives on human illness for which there is no cure, today's victims of arthritis and related diseases—more than 37 million Americans, according to the Arthritis Foundation—continue to be prime targets of hucksters, miracle-cure promoters, and charlatans. A nonprofit national health organization, the Arthritis Foundation estimates that the annual U.S. bill for unproven or quack arthritis remedies is over a billion dollars.

Fortunately, many arthritis victims who once would have faced the prospect of chronic pain and eventual disability can now be helped by a number of drugs and surgical techniques. But quackery has kept pace. In fact, the foundation believes that far more money is spent on worthless nostrums than for scientific research about arthritic diseases.

For some patients, the outlay for various food supplements, wonder-diet books, folk remedies, liniments, and miracle devices is merely a waste of money. For others, however, the consequences are more serious. Some quack regimens are inherently unsafe—direct hazards. Others are indirect hazards—though innocuous in themselves, they may lead people to delay seeking proper treatment or to abandon medically prescribed therapy.

Early diagnosis and sustained treatment may prevent much of the pain and disability caused by rheumatoid arthritis, yet many people with this condition wait months or even years before seeking medical help. Often a factor in such delay is reliance on self-medication with over-the-counter products, home remedies, and the offerings of quacks. Ignorance about arthritis—and what should and should not be done for it—can be a serious handicap.

Many Causes and Types of Arthritis

The word *arthritis* literally means "inflammation of a joint." But arthritis is actually many diseases—some mild, some severe. More than 100 different ailments come under the heading of arthritis (or "rheumatism," a term sometimes used for unexplained aches and pains). Symptomatically, all of them are characterized by pain in the joints and muscles. The more severe forms also show overt evidence of inflammation (redness, heat, and swelling) as well as pain, and some forms may affect other parts of the body besides the joints and muscles.

The various types of arthritis can be differentiated from one another. The course of each of the forms of arthritis is variable—a fact that purveyors of catchall remedies commonly ignore. Some types of arthritis arise from still unexplained inflammatory processes. Others are caused by the degenerative effects of aging, by severe or repeated injury to a joint, or even by certain infections.

For most forms of arthritis, there is no cure. But many types can be controlled, and their effects minimized, by proper treatment. The most important step in the control process is diagnosing the specific form of arthritis involved—as early as possible—so that treatment can begin before permanent damage occurs.

The most widespread kind of arthritis is osteoarthritis, or degenerative joint disease. Although sometimes the cause of acute joint inflammation, it is primarily a "wear-and-tear" disease. Most frequently it affects the large weight-bearing joints, such as the hips and knees, often causing pain on walking. Approximately 16 million people in the United States require some medical care for osteoarthritis. Although the ailment is usually mild, it can be severe. Nearly all people get at least a touch of osteoarthritis if they live long enough.

The second most common joint disease, according to the Arthritis Foundation, is rheumatoid arthritis, an inflammatory condition now estimated to affect more than two million adults. It tends to be a recurrent process, causing pain, swelling, and, in some cases, deformities in many joints, especially in the knuckles and middle joint of the fingers. Rheumatoid arthritis usually starts between ages twenty and forty-five, affecting about three times as many women as men. A similar disease, juvenile rheumatoid arthritis, can begin at any age from infancy through the teens.

In both the adult and childhood forms, medical treatment can usually relieve symptoms and minimize disability. And the severe disabilities that do occur can sometimes be helped by surgery. Nevertheless, people with rheumatoid arthritis often are easy targets for quacks. One reason is that the disorder is subject to periods of remission during which pain spontaneously subsides and symptoms disappear. If the improvement happens to coincide with the use of an unconventional remedy, the patient may think the treatment cured the disease. Such experiences are the basis of many sincere testimonials for worthless products or therapies.

The third most frequent arthritic ailment is gout, which affects about one million people, the majority of them men. Its acute form commonly strikes the large joint of the big toe, but it can also start in the knee, ankle, or other large joints. The course of gout can vary from a few attacks in a lifetime to a progressive disease that begins at puberty and can cripple its victims by the age of forty if untreated. Gout can also cause kidney stones in some patients. Fortunately, modern therapy can relieve or prevent both the joint and kidney manifestations and can virtually eliminate the danger of crippling.

Among other forms of arthritis, two are most prevalent. One is ankylosing spondylitis, an inflammation that commonly strikes males during their teens or twenties, and which results in stiffness and sometimes deformity of the spine. Also called Marie-Strumpell's disease, it affects 1.3 people per thousand. Another type of arthritis that occurs with about half this frequency is systemic lupus erythematosus, which can affect the skin and internal organs as well as the joints. Most of the victims are women. Commonly called "lupus," the disease usually can be controlled, although in severe cases, usually involving the kidneys, it can be life threatening.

Even a brief rundown of the major types of arthritis reveals one obvious fact: joint pain can mean any number of things. An aching knee might arise from a simple sprain or from bursitis, osteoarthritis, gout, or a related disease. It could stem from a wear-and-tear process or be an indication of a more generalized disease. Some patients experience joint pain that defies quick analysis.

Beyond diagnosis, the treatment for a specific disease can vary considerably from person to person. One arthritis patient may respond well to a particular drug, but another with the same illness may gain only marginal relief or experience intolerable side effects. In short, the diagnosis and treatment of arthritic diseases can be a complicated process, often requiring patience and cooperation on the part of both the patient and the physician.

"Quick and Easy" Solutions

In contrast, unproven or irrational methods are usually hawked as panaceas to all comers. Such answers to pain and crippling are available to anyone willing to spend the money for a convenient bottle, a dietary supplement touted by a book, a magazine or newspaper article, a radio "authority," or a clinic offering a secret or miraculous cure. It sometimes seems as though every type of offbeat treatment has been promoted for arthritis. The gimmicks have run the gamut from copper bracelets, venoms, and "immune" milk to mechanical contraptions, radioactive pads, "moon dust," and potent drugs.

Arthritis sufferers are good customers for such items. A 1986 FDA-sponsored survey of 247 people diagnosed with arthritis found that 24 percent considered their condition serious or very serious. Eighteen percent said they almost always had a significant amount of pain, while another 22 percent said that their condition frequently caused significant pain. About one out of three said they would be willing to try anything for their condition even if it sounds silly or has a small probability of success. And about the same percentage said they had tried at least one of the questionable methods listed in the survey. The most frequently tried methods were vitamins (17 percent), vibrators (14 percent), special diets (12 percent), chiropractic (12 percent), alfalfa tablets (9 percent), copper bracelets (9 percent), honey/vinegar (8 percent), and cod liver or fish oil (8 percent).

Jerry Walsh, who at age eighteen was stricken with rheumatoid arthritis, later spent many years crusading against quackery for the Arthritis Foundation. Once, following a television appearance, he received 5,700 letters. More than 80 percent of them were from arthritis victims who asked where they could obtain one or more of the fake treatments he had just exposed! Walsh was startled but understood what had produced the avalanche of mail. During the early years of his illness, he himself had wasted thousands of dollars on quack remedies.

When Walsh appeared before the U.S. Senate Special Committee on Aging in 1963, he eloquently recounted what arthritic pain can mean:

> I can guarantee any of you gentlemen . . . that if you are in this bed of pain with arthritis, you will try anything to stop the pain, at any cost. You say, "What have you got to lose?" I know that I went from copper bracelets to buckeyes trying to find a cure. I've tried vibrating machines and diets, and

had a chiropractor break one of my legs with his special treatment. Yet, continually, I went back, maybe to the tune of $2,000 or $3,000 more. You don't keep track of the dollars, and in fact you like to forget them. You are always looking for relief. . . . If someone would approach me today offering me, with a glib tongue and all, the opportunity of getting better . . . I am sure that I would think it over maybe for a couple of days. If I could do it in the back room unbeknown to you gentlemen, and I wouldn't have much to lose in time or money— and I don't know where I would draw the line . . . $200 or $300—I am sure that I would sneak a treatment.

Mechanical Devices

Years ago, mechanical devices were the prime staple of arthritis quackery. Priced at $9.95, the *Miracle Health Relaxer* was promised to relieve both arthritis and constipation. A *Vrilium Tube* cost a bit more; it contained 2¢ worth of salt and sold for $250. By contrast, the *Vivicosmic Disk* was a bargain— only $5 for a piece of cement. Among the most popular devices were vibrators. A certain model for arthritics came with five attachments, including one guaranteed to banish dandruff. And there was the *Pulse-A-Rhythm* vibrating mattress, marketed until the FDA seized the product, calling it ineffective and dangerous for those it was touted to help.

Radiation

For a while, radiation was in vogue. Arthritis victims could pay for the privilege of sitting in an abandoned uranium mine to absorb the "healing radiations" of radon. If they were too poor or too crippled to take advantage of this sovereign remedy, they could still buy mitts or pads supposedly containing low-grade radioactive ore. A typical one, the Marvpad, cost $30 and was filled with gravel. Most such gimmicks have now faded from the marketplace, according to the Arthritis Foundation. Today, the emphasis in arthritis promotions is mainly on diet and nutrition.

Diet and Dietary Supplements

Worthless diet cures have always been a part of arthritis mythology. If the magic nutrient wasn't cod liver oil, it might have been alfalfa or pokeberries or Honegar—the mixture concocted by the late D. D. Jarvis, M.D., out of honey and vinegar plus a bit of iodine and kelp. In recent years there has been a virtual bandwagon of public interest in many aspects of nutrition, including claims of attaining "superhealth" at the dinner table. Arthritis-cure promoters have been quick to join the parade, and various arthritis diet books have flourished.

When *The Arthritic's Cookbook* sold well, out came a sequel, *New Hope for the Arthritic* (touting the same diet). If the appetite was satisfied but the joints still ached, another heavily advertised candidate, *A Doctor's Proven New Home Cure for Arthritis*, could be tried. No relief? Perhaps *There Is a Cure for Arthritis* would hit on the right menu.

Another popular book has been Dale Alexander's *Arthritis and Common Sense*, which has reportedly sold over a million copies. Alexander—who is sometimes referred to as "the Codfather"—claims that the basic cause of arthritis is "poorly lubricated joints" and that dietary oils (particularly cod liver oil) relieve arthritis by lubricating the joints. This claim is obviously false—no *oil* taken orally can ever wind up in a body joint! Those oils are broken down by digestion into simple substances before absorption from the intestinal tract. In a recently published interview, Alexander said that arthritics should allow at least six months to assess the results of taking cod liver oil because "it could take that long for the whole body to lubricate itself." That, of course, would be sufficient time for some arthritics to undergo spontaneous improvement—for which Alexander would no doubt like to claim credit.

Health food industry manufacturers market a steady stream of dietary supplements touted for arthritis. Since it would be illegal to market them with therapeutic claims—unless approved by the FDA—many of these products have no claim on their label but just list the ingredients. Some manufacturers choose product names (such as *Artho Tabs* and *Ar Pak*) to suggest effectiveness against arthritis. Others, playing it safer, market substances labeled mucopolysaccharides or evening primrose oil, relying on publications, talk show guests, and health food retailers to convey what the substances are supposed to do.

The truth is that there's little or no scientific evidence that any food or vitamin has much to do with causing or curing arthritis. "The proper diet for someone with arthritis," advises the Arthritis Foundation, "is a normal, well-balanced, nourishing diet—the same things people without arthritis should eat. The one exception is with gouty arthritis. Certain foods—primarily organ meats such as liver and kidney—may increase uric acid levels in the blood and should be avoided." Some arthritis victims who are overweight may need a reducing diet to ease the burden on weight-bearing joints. But, otherwise, diet regimens touted for arthritis are about as useful as the *Pulse-A-Rhythm* mattress or the *Vivicosmic Disk*.

Other Offbeat Approaches

Over the years, any number of doctors have publicized off-beat remedies for arthritis. If the regimens later proved to be ineffective, they often fell by the wayside. But not always. A physician's faith in the remedy—or faith in its money-making potential—could help generate enough publicity to keep it alive. And any remedy, no matter how controversial, can seem inviting to an arthritis victim in chronic pain.

Among the holdovers still attracting attention is dimethyl sulfoxide (DMSO). The FDA has approved its use for only one disease: interstitial cystitis, an uncommon bladder disorder. It has not been demonstrated to provide long-term benefit for any form of rheumatic disease, and reputable physicians don't prescribe it (see page 66).

Procaine preparations, sometimes sold under the names GH3 or Gerovital H3, have been promoted for arthritis pain. Sellers of these quack nostrums have claimed they also provide relief for angina, deafness, senile psychosis, and impotence. Procaine is a local anesthetic and in slightly altered form is useful against heart rhythm disturbance. But it has no value in the treatment of any other conditions.

Meanwhile, alleged breakthroughs in arthritis treatment continue to be heralded from time to time in the media. Arthritis has been reported to be an allergic disease that could be alleviated by a starvation diet. Some 500 arthritis patients were said to have improved dramatically after treatment with a flu vaccine. Arthritis patients were supposedly helped by taking tablets derived from yucca plants. Invariably, when Arthritis Foundation specialists investigated these reports, they found no scientific evidence to back up the claims.

More Dangerous Approaches

Cortisone and similar steroid drugs can provide dramatic reduction of pain and inflammation in a matter of hours or days. But daily use of steroids for prolonged periods can cause serious side effects, particularly at high dosage levels. These effects can sometimes be more severe than the arthritis, and even life threatening. Accordingly, while steroids and other potent drugs still have a valuable place in arthritis treatment, their use is commonly reserved only for severe cases where the benefits outweigh the risks.

In recent decades, however, a few physicians have gained notoriety and wealth by dispensing large quantities of steroid concoctions and other potentially dangerous drugs. Lured by the hope of a cure, thousands of patients have traveled to clinics in Canada, the Dominican Republic, or Mexico, to obtain such drugs as *Liefcort*, *Rheumatril*, DMSO, or unnamed "secret" remedies.

Arthritis and the Popular Press

Arthritis-cure promoters know the importance of publicity and are often skillful at using the media to their advantage. In 1962, Liefcort became a smashing success on the strength of one national magazine story. But arthritis can be a money-maker for the media as well. A potential market of 37 million sufferers makes arthritis a prime topic for publications that trade in sensationalism, particularly some of the "checkout counter" tabloids. In recent years, for example, the front page of the *National Examiner* called attention to "New Ways to Banish Arthritis and Headaches," "Nature's Miracle Cures for Arthritis and High Blood Pressure," "New Diet to Ease Pain of Arthritis," and "How to Wash Away Arthritis Pain Instantly," while the *Sun*'s front page proclaimed that "Miracle Caves Cure Thousands of Arthritis."

Articles of this type tend to fall into three categories: (1) sensationalized presentations of useful methods known well to arthritis victims; (2) preliminary reports of research findings that have no practical significance; and (3) one-sided reports touting quack nonsense. Among the above articles: the "new ways to banish arthritis" were based on the notion that arthritis is caused by food allergies; the "miracle cure" was fruits that supposedly rid the body of toxins that cause arthritis; the "new diet" was a standard low-fat, high-fiber diet plus vitamin supplements; the way to "wash away pain instantly" was a hot bath; and the "miracle caves" were tunnels in the uranium mines mentioned earlier in this chapter.

Health food magazines such as *Let's Live* and *Bestways* also promote vitamin and mineral supplements as arthritis remedies.

Over-the-Counter Hype

Some reputable over-the-counter (OTC) drug manufacturers are not averse to cashing in on arthritic discomfort. Most OTC pain-relievers contain one of three basic ingredients: aspirin, acetaminophen, and ibuprofen. Each is available in low-cost generic versions, as well as in many higher-cost brand-name compounds. Small doses of any of these may be effective against the aches and pains of mild forms of arthritis. So-called arthritis-strength tablets are a bit larger, contain a bit more drug per tablet, and may contain some antacid, but they are essentially expensive forms of their lower-dose counterparts.

In higher doses, aspirin and ibuprofen can be effective against arthritic *inflammation*, but high doses should be administered under the guidance of a physician. In fact, CU's medical consultants point out, consumers who self-treat arthritis symptoms with an OTC pain-reliever without medical supervision may be risking irreversible damage to joints (in addition to serious side effects)—damage that might be preventable with optimum treatment.

Liniments, ointments, and body rubs are also heavily promoted for relief of arthritis aches and pains. These OTC products depend on one or more skin irritants for their effect— usually methyl salicylate (oil of wintergreen) and various combinations of others. When massaged onto the skin, they tend to increase blood flow in the upper layers, resulting in slight reddening as well as a sensation of warmth. The mild increase in skin temperature—as well as any muscle relaxation induced by the massage—may provide brief symptomatic relief, but a warm bath would probably be at least as effective.

Proper Diagnosis and Treatment

About one out of every six visits to a family physician or internist is for problems involving muscles, joints, tendons, or ligaments. Many such ailments involve localized muscle pain or some other self-limited symptom that will clear up in a few days even without treatment. All that may be needed is rest and a mild pain medication. But claims for unproven or quack arthritis remedies are frequently based on "successful" treatment of just such complaints.

If pain in one or more joints is accompanied by fever, persists for a week or two, or recurs over a period of weeks, a physician should be consulted. Gonorrhea, gout, rheumatoid arthritis, and occasionally osteoarthritis may begin as an acute inflammatory arthritis, with redness, heat, pain, and swelling of the involved joint. Such symptoms usually prompt the victim to seek immediate medical attention. More often, though, arthritis symptoms come on gradually. The symptoms may appear for a few days and go away, then come back stronger and disappear again. There may be weeks or months between goings and comings, but gradually the disease reappears at shorter intervals until it becomes a daily problem that is more difficult to ignore.

Flare-ups and remissions are common in rheumatoid arthritis, ankylosing spondylitis, and other inflammatory arthritic diseases. Consequently, any recurring joint symptom should be checked with a doctor, no matter how mild or "temporary" it might appear at first. Physical examination, X-ray films, and specific laboratory tests can help distinguish arthritis from less serious ailments and differentiate one type of arthritis from another. Sometimes examination of the joint fluid is also necessary. The sooner the ailment is diagnosed and treatment begins, the greater the likelihood of lessening permanent joint damage.

Although there is still no cure, prospects have greatly improved for arthritis victims. With early diagnosis and treatment, many can now minimize disability and lead a relatively normal life. Current therapy includes medications, exercise, and other physical measures. In cases of severe joint damage, surgery may be utilized. Individual treatment varies widely, depending on the type of arthritis, its severity, and the patient's response to therapy.

Medication Without Hype

Drug therapy is the first line of defense against arthritis. In most cases its immediate goal is to reduce inflammation and pain. Ultimately, the objective is to preserve joint function. The reduction in pain and swelling helps the patient maintain joint mobility, which might otherwise not be possible. The anti-inflammatory effect also serves to minimize or prevent joint damage.

The most frequently prescribed drug for arthritis is aspirin. Its familiarity as a household remedy for headaches or minor aches and pains often makes people doubt that aspirin can work effectively against serious forms of arthritis. But it can. In large doses, commonly 10 to 15 five-grain tablets daily, aspirin is often effective in suppressing joint inflammation, and it is the mainstay for many arthritis patients. It is not, however, a perfect drug. People vary in their tolerance for aspirin, and some cannot take it at all. Large doses may cause stomach irritation and bleeding, which can be mild or severe. Other common side effects include ringing in the ears and temporary hearing loss. To control such effects, physicians may reduce the dosage, prescribe enteric-coated aspirin, or try other salicylate drugs similar to aspirin.

Some patients, however, may not get adequate relief from salicylates. Nor are these drugs effective in all arthritic disorders. In the treatment of acute gout, for example, aspirin has no place (small doses may increase uric acid in the blood and aggravate the condition), and physicians may prescribe another anti-inflammatory agent or colchicine, a gout-specific medication used for decades for this purpose. In infectious types of arthritis, the early use of antibiotics can spell the difference between cure and a chronically stiff, deformed joint. For a person with osteoarthritis and rheumatoid arthritis, however, finding the right drug can be an extended process of trial and error, starting with the safest drugs that are likely to be of benefit and moving up to riskier ones if necessary. Several drugs may be evaluated, in varying doses, until the best one is found.

Many nonsteroidal anti-inflammatory drugs (NSAIDS) offer

alternatives for individualized therapy. These drugs include ibuprofen (*Motrin*), naproxen (*Naprosyn*), diclofenac (*Voltarin*), and a score of others. In appropriate dosage, they are comparable to aspirin in anti-inflammatory effect, and for some patients their side effects seem milder than those from high doses of aspirin—though they still can cause serious gastrointestinal symptoms such as bleeding and ulceration. All are far more expensive than aspirin, and all except ibuprofen in low dosage require a doctor's prescription.

If a patient doesn't respond adequately to aspirin or other NSAIDS, other drugs may be used. All involve a greater risk of serious side effects than the initial group of drugs. But they can be helpful to patients who might not otherwise obtain relief.

Drug therapy for rheumatoid arthritis has been evolving rapidly. Gold salts (injectable and oral) and penicillamine have been joined by hydroxychloroquine (Plaquenil) (an antimalarial drug), methotrexate (a chemotherapeutic agent used against cancer), sulfasalazine (a drug used for treating inflammatory bowel disease), azathioprine and cyclophosphamide (immunosuppressive drugs), and a host of other "secondline" drugs. Unlike aspirin and other NSAIDS, these drugs do not provide immediate pain relief, but they may delay progression of the disease or allow reduction in dosage of other drugs that have more side effects.

Cortisone-related steroids, such as prednisone, are another class of drugs that must be used with caution. Although they can provide dramatic relief of pain and swelling in inflamed joints, their numerous side effects limit their usefulness in prolonged therapy. Unlike gold salts and penicillamine, which some patients can tolerate well for years, steroids eventually produce serious side effects in all patients during extended therapy, unless given in very low dosage. Accordingly, in certain cases when oral steroids are the only alternative, they are generally used in the smallest amounts that will improve symptoms—sometimes on an every-other-day basis. Direct injection of steroids into a particularly painful joint is still a common method of relief and is relatively free of hazard if used infrequently.

Physical Measures

While medication is the cornerstone of arthritis treatment, physical measures are also important. Part of the goal is to achieve a proper balance between rest and exercise. During a flare-up, rest can be as important as medication. Complete body rest is rarely needed, but exercise of any affected "hot" joints should be minimized to help reduce inflammation and prevent further damage. Heat treatment, such as hot soaks, baths, and showers, are commonly prescribed to relieve pain and stiffness. Frequently, a patient will respond better to cold packs around an acutely inflamed joint than to heat. Whirlpool baths or other forms of hydrotherapy may also be useful. Individual joints are sometimes rested in removable, lightweight splints. That helps lessen inflammation and keeps the joint in a normal-use position, protecting it against muscle flexion deformities (contractures) that might lead to permanent disfigurement. Splints may also be used to help straighten out a joint that has become fixed in a flexed position. The splints are usually adjusted every few days to move the joint toward the desired position.

Once inflammation and pain subside, more emphasis is placed on exercise. For arthritis patients, exercise does not mean engaging in athletics or similarly strenuous activities. It involves putting joints gently through their full range of motion every day. This helps maintain normal joint movement and helps strengthen muscles that may have been weakened by inactivity. As joint function improves, the exercises may be done against slight resistance—provided there is no pain. Generally, each patient requires an individually prescribed program of exercises. Occupational therapy can often help patients master the tasks of everyday living despite painful disabilities.

An appropriate program of rest and exercise that is followed faithfully not only may prevent deformities but also may help correct those that might already have developed. One problem, however, is that some patients who feel better forgo their exercises and even their medication. The result may be an earlier or more severe return of symptoms than might otherwise occur.

Since the early 1960s, when the first successful total hip joint replacement was performed, numerous surgical techniques have been developed to undo the crippling effects of arthritis. Total hip replacement represents one of the major advances in orthopedic surgery of the past century. The knee joint—a common site of arthritic damage—can also be replaced with artificial components. And similar operations for the hand, wrist, elbow, ankle, and shoulder are being performed. Complications or failure can occur with any of the operations, and not every patient with a severe disability is a candidate for joint replacement. But for many patients, these operations—as well as several other types—can relieve pain, correct deformities, and improve joint function. To a large extent, the success of joint surgery depends on the patient's willingness to participate actively in a postoperative therapy program that may be prolonged. Appropriate exercise is essential to gain function and strength in the reconstructed parts. Without such effort, the best surgical procedures may fail.

Where to Get Help

When people first seek medical help for arthritis symptoms, they ordinarily turn to a family physician or internist. When diagnosis and treatment of the more serious forms of arthritis require specialized knowledge, the patient may be referred to a rheumatologist, a nonsurgical specialist in arthritic diseases. The Arthritis Foundation, which can provide literature and supply the names of qualified rheumatologists, has local chapters in more than 70 American cities. If no chapter is listed in your local telephone directory, write to the foundation at P.O. Box 19000, Atlanta, Georgia 30326. Additional information can be obtained from several books on the recommended reading list in Appendix 3.

9

Weight Control:
Fads and Fakes

Humorist Art Buchwald suggested that the word *diet* comes from the verb *to die*. Anyone whose commitment to weight loss has fallen victim to hunger pangs, headaches, fatigue, dizziness, or just plain boredom might well agree. Most overweight people have discovered that losing weight—and maintaining the loss—is no easy matter. The frequent failure of low-calorie diets and "willpower" to overcome obesity has spawned a profusion of fad diets, "magic" pills, and quack gadgets. Most of these measures slenderize only one's bank account, but some can introduce health complications of their own.

Despite the realities, the promise of a new or effortless way to lose weight often attracts attention quickly. Many magazines carry frequent articles touting the latest wonder diet. Readers disillusioned with the grapefruit diet or the drinking man's diet, weary of bouncing from a vegetarian diet to a Stone Age diet, or from a gourmet diet to a brown bag diet, can still try their luck with a 30-day countdown diet, a nine-day wonder diet, or a 24-hour easy diet. When those fail, dieters can eat themselves slim—and fat again—the French way, seek solace in the pray-your-weight diet, or turn to a wide array of books promoting equally foolproof schemes.

Fad diet books typically have several things in common. They claim to offer a revolutionary new idea based on the author's personal experience. They suggest that certain nutrients, foods, or food combinations are either the key to weight reduction or villains that prevent it. And they present information—much of it inaccurate—about the biochemistry of weight control. Many fad diets are nutritionally unbalanced.

During the past two decades, many best-selling diet plans have emphasized proteins, some recommending "unlimited" amounts and others calling for small amounts. Food combination schemes have also achieved notoriety.

Modified Fasting

The concept of the very-low-calorie (VLC) diet evolved from research in the 1970s with an approach called the "protein-sparing modified fast." This was not a diet for the general public, but a hospital-based program for extremely obese patients whose weight problem was considered life threatening.

Participation was limited to the massively obese because fasting is potentially dangerous. After several days on a total fast, the body begins to burn not only its fat stores but protein tissue as well. And that protein comes from lean body mass— muscles and major organs such as the heart and kidneys. Prolonged fasting can also lead to anemia, impairment of liver function, gall bladder and kidney stones, mineral imbalances, and other problems. As with many diets, the modified fast produces weight loss due to loss of body water (dehydration), particularly during the first few days. But this component of weight loss is illusory. As soon as the dieter resumes a more balanced diet, the weight lost through dehydration is regained.

The aim of the modified fast is to supply just enough protein or other nourishment to prevent the body from cannibalizing its own lean tissue. This approach was viewed by its originators as relatively severe but justified in cases where the potential benefits outweighed the risks. It was not simply a diet but included intensive supervision to help the participants make permanent changes in their eating habits and life-style. Once the early results were in, however, it didn't take long for entrepreneurs to begin promoting similar plans for the "do-it-yourself" dieter.

The Last Chance Diet, by Robert Linn, D.O., was touted as the diet of choice "when everything else fails." Published in 1976, the regimen consisted of only a few ounces of liquid protein daily plus vitamin and mineral supplements and non-caloric drinks. The book quickly hit the best-seller list and stimulated a flood of protein supplements. But tragedy soon followed. Whereas the supervised VLC research programs had used high-quality protein, Linn's regimen and many of its imitators did not. As a result, many people became ill, and more than 39 deaths occurred, probably as a result of sudden disturbances of heart rhythm.

Today, modified fasting has been "legitimized" for outpatient treatment under medical supervision. But a recent editorial in the *Journal of the American Medical Association* (January 5, 1990) warned that popularization of VLC diets—by such events as Oprah Winfrey's celebrated 67-pound weight loss—could lead to dangerous misuse. Experts fear that the vigorous marketing of meal-replacement drinks will encourage people to use these products without adequate medical supervision. The more meals replaced and the lower the number of calories consumed daily, the greater the risk. The risk is greatest in individuals who are *not* severely overweight. The FDA now requires a warning label on weight-reduction products when more than half of their calories come from protein.

VLC diets commonly contain 600 to 800 calories per day, most of them from high-quality proteins, plus vitamins and minerals, particularly potassium. Some programs use liquid formulas, whereas others utilize food sources (poultry, fish, and lean meats). Experts believe that diets this drastic should be restricted to individuals who are at least 30 percent overweight and should be administered only under close medical supervision as part of a comprehensive program. Such a program should include a weekly examination by a physician familiar with the metabolic effects of VLC diets, blood tests to detect potentially dangerous metabolic abnormalities, and behavior modification therapy. Even so, once the eating of food is resumed, weight gain is common (though perhaps not as common as with do-it-yourself efforts).

High-Protein Diets

In the 1976 edition of *The Health Robbers*, Jean Mayer, Ph.D., noted that the high-protein (low-carbohydrate) diet first appeared in the 1860s as the Banting diet and reappeared in modern times as the Du Pont diet, the Johns Hopkins diet (disavowed by Johns Hopkins Medical School), the Mayo Clinic diet (disavowed by the Mayo Clinic), the Stillman Doctor's Quick Weight-Loss diet (which included eight glasses of water per day), and a host of other names. One of the best known and most extreme forms was described in 1971 by

Robert Atkins, M.D., in his book *Dr. Atkins' Diet Revolution*. All these diet plans restrict sugars and starches.

Promoters of high-protein diets claim that altering the proportions of fats, proteins, and carbohydrates in the diet leads to increased metabolism of unwanted fat whether or not calories are restricted. Actually, there is no evidence that unbalancing the diet will have any metabolic effect that speeds or slows the loss of body fat. Yet weight loss often occurs because obese individuals who drastically reduce their carbohydrate intake are apparently unable to compensate by increasing their intake of protein and fat—as a result of the diet's monotony. Thus, mainly because fewer calories are consumed, weight loss occurs. As with fasting diets, low-carbohydrate diets can cause the body to burn fat and protein tissue, with similar health hazards. And, since meats tend to be high in both saturated fat and cholesterol, unrestricted high-protein diets can be dangerous, especially for people whose blood cholesterol levels are already high.

Sheer Nonsense

It would be difficult to choose the most ridiculous diet book ever written—there are so many candidates—but surely *Fit for Life*, by "Dr." Harvey Diamond and his wife, Marilyn, would be right up there.

Published in 1986, *Fit for Life* is based on the notion that when certain foods are combined in the body, they "rot and putrefy," creating digestive cesspools that somehow poison the system and make a person fat. To avoid this, the authors recommend that fats, carbohydrates, and protein foods be eaten at separate meals, concentrating on fruits in the morning and vegetables in the afternoon. They favor fruits and vegetables, they say, because foods high in water content can "wash the toxic from the inside of the body" instead of "clogging" the body.

Actually, digestion is a process of controlled rot and decay in which digestive juices break down the foods into smaller chemical components so they can pass through the intestinal wall. Contrary to the Diamonds' assertion, the process is completed without "clogging" within a few hours.

Neither of the authors of *Fit for Life* had scientific training in nutrition. Harvey's "Ph.D. in nutritional science" was obtained from the American College of Health Science, a correspondence school in Texas that teaches the philosophy of the late Herbert Shelton, founder of "Natural Hygiene." The school not only was unaccredited but lacked authorization from the state to grant degrees. In 1987, the school's president, T. C. Fry, agreed to a permanent injunction barring him from issuing more "degrees" and even from calling his operation a college.

In 1986 Katherine Musgrave, Ph.D., a professor of nutrition at the University of Maine, used a computer to analyze seven days of menus printed in *Fit for Life*. She found that the diet was marginal in iron and deficient in zinc, calcium, vitamin D, and vitamin B_{12}. Over a period of several weeks, these shortages are unlikely to cause trouble. But as a lifelong program (which the authors recommend), the diet could result in significant deficiencies.

Despite its nonsense, the book was a great commercial success. Television appearances on the Merv Griffin and Donahue shows helped generate sales of more than a million copies. Commenting on this, Dr. William Jarvis, president of the National Council Against Health Fraud, stated:

Fit for Life seems unprecedented in the amount of misinformation contained. It is appalling that such a book can become a best seller in the latter half of the 20th century. Its only socially redeeming feature is that its popularity may alert American educators to their failure to impart the most fundamental knowledge about health and nutrition to the students entrusted to their care.

Dubious Devices

The battle of the bulge is also being fought in another arena, with mechanical and electrical devices arrayed in slenderizing salons, gymnasiums, and health clubs. Various devices may provide passive exercise, vibration, or massage. Although these devices and the methods of using them differ, they do have two things in common. First, they are promoted primarily in terms of girth reduction rather than weight reduction. Second, they don't work.

It is a sad but simple fact that the only way to slenderize a body part is to lose weight overall. Then the fat deposits throughout the body will decrease according to one's hereditary makeup. No benefit is likely to accrue from "passive exercise."

Electrical muscle stimulators—also called EMS devices—are claimed to contour the body by delivering low-voltage electric shocks. Promoters of these devices allege that an overweight person's muscles are soft and flabby and that stimulating them to contract by means of electrical impulses improves their tone and causes them to shrink. However, the muscles of a fat person are overlaid with fat and not necessarily soft—

as some professional football players demonstrate. Electrical stimulation could conceivably cause a muscle to enlarge, but it can't affect the overlying fat. Some EMS devices play a legitimate role in physical therapy; they can be used to help prevent blood clots or retard muscle wasting in paralyzed muscles. But no such device can reshape the body, remove wrinkles, enlarge the bust, or provide any other cosmetic benefit. Worse yet, EMS devices can cause electrical shocks and burns if they are used incorrectly or have not been manufactured properly.

Motor-driven rowing machines or bicyclelike devices yield the benefits of exercise in proportion to the amount of effort that goes into the movements. Merely relaxing on the machine and letting it pull the body through the motions may be soothing—like a massage—and may contribute slightly to improved muscle tone. Real exercise, however, requires the use of a machine without a motor.

Perhaps the most common devices promoted for the overweight are vibrators—everything from elaborate tables, couches, chairs, and beds to cushions, belts, and small handheld appliances at prices ranging from a few dollars to several hundred. The vibrations of some of the larger devices cause passive body movements by means of rhythmic, rocking motions. What value there is in such motions is not known, but it is incorrect to assert, as has been done, that 45 minutes on a rocking table is equivalent to playing 36 holes of golf or horseback riding 10 miles at a canter. The motion may be relaxing or soothing, but it cannot produce weight loss.

With most other devices the vibrations are faster and the movements smaller. Some promoters claim that their products (sometimes together with a diet plan) will break down fat, produce a firmer, more graceful figure, provide "exercise without effort," and relieve tension and fatigue. Some have even risked legal difficulties with government regulatory agencies, claiming effectiveness against arthritis pain, menstrual cramps, backaches, headaches, and high blood pressure.

Claims that vibrators are effective in promoting weight reduction or treating disease are false and misleading. But to the degree that the devices may produce effects similar to those provided by classic massage techniques, some of the less innocuous claims may have a certain basis in fact. Massage has been used since ancient times to soothe tired, painful joints and muscles and to induce relaxation. Massage causes a slight increase in surface blood flow and skin temperature.

This, however, is far from saying that the use of a vibrating bed, pillow, abdominal belt, or other device will "tone up" muscles and reduce girth. Nor will massage remove fat deposits under the skin, whether done by hand, vibrator device, or the mechanical rollers that pound the hips of people in television commercials. Studies have shown, for example, that massage of an arm and a leg produced no significant decrease in girth when compared with the unmassaged arm and leg of the same person. In test subjects who were simultaneously dieting, decrease in girth was approximately the same in both limbs.

Many wearable products have been promoted for weight reduction, including so-called sauna shorts and belts, body wraps dipped in chemical solutions, and others. All are ineffective at best, and some are downright dangerous. Body wraps can be hazardous for people suffering from diabetes or diseases of the arteries and veins of the legs.

Pills and Potions

The desperate can also try pills "guaranteed" to produce rapid and permanent weight loss by altering the absorption or metabolism of foods. Dozens of such pills are offered each year through direct-mail solicitations and newspaper advertising, most notably in the tabloids.

Some of these pills, as well as others sold over-the-counter, contain phenylpropanolamine (PPA), a nasal decongestant that has a temporary effect on appetite in some people. But— as noted in the November 1989 *Consumer Reports Health Letter*—there is no evidence that their use has any long-term benefit for weight control. Moreover, there is a narrow margin between so-called safe use and amounts that can cause side effects, including an increase in blood pressure.

Other mail-order pills have been claimed to block the absorption of starch, fat, or calories, to flush fat out of the body, or to step up the body's "fat-burning system." These claims have no factual basis.

Some diet pills contain a fiber, such as glucomannan or guar gum, that is claimed to curb appetite by absorbing water and swelling to fill the stomach. This claim is false. The amount of fiber is too small to actually fill the stomach, and even if it could, that would not necessarily curb a person's appetite. Moreover, double-blind tests have shown that so-called bulking agents don't result in weight loss.

In July 1990, government enforcement agencies ended the sale of *Cal-Ban 3000*, a guar gum product that had been claimed to produce automatic weight loss without dieting or exercise. Postal authorities secured a temporary injunction. Florida officials filed civil and criminal complaints (later settled for penalties totaling $1,305,000), and the FDA requested a recall. The FDA said that health professionals had reported 17 cases of people who experienced esophageal obstruction after ingesting *Cal-Ban* tablets, which swell to several times their size when wet. Ten of these people were hospitalized, and one died.

Some diet products contain benzocaine, a topical anesthetic

claimed to decrease appetite by diminishing the sense of taste. But there is no convincing evidence that benzocaine is effective in long-term weight reduction.

Among the products analyzed by CU medical consultants during the past few years, the following have been marketed with false, misleading, or exaggerated claims.

Spirulina, a dark-green powder or pill derived from algae, is said by its promoters to suppress appetite. However, there is no scientific evidence to support this claim. Products containing *Gymnema sylvestre* are being touted as weight-control aids with claims that they block the absorption of sugar. The leaves of this plant, when chewed, can prevent the taste sensation of sweetness. But there is no evidence that *Gymnema sylvestre* blocks absorption of sugar into the body. A number of prescription drugs are being marketed as weight-control aids. Most experts believe that amphetamines should not be used for weight control because they are addictive and unsafe. (Fenfluramine and various other drugs might be appropriate for carefully selected people as part of a comprehensive medically supervised research program, but side effects are common, and little scientific data supports their use.) Diuretics ("water pills") are sometimes prescribed as part of a weight-loss program. This practice is irrational because any weight lost in this manner will quickly return when the diuretic wears off and the body is rehydrated.

The "Simple" Facts

Under ordinary circumstances, an adult whose weight is about right should eat the kind and amounts of food that permit maintaining that weight with little or no gain or loss. Beyond these minor fluctuations, if weight should begin to rise or is already too high, it is time to cut down on total calorie intake and increase calorie expenditure. The whole problem of weight control is as simple—or as difficult—as that.

To lose a pound of body weight, a dieter must eliminate about 3,500 calories. For example, if current daily intake totals 2,700 calories, and this daily intake is lowered by 500 calories to 2,200 calories per day, weight loss theoretically should proceed at the rate of one pound per week—assuming all other variables remain stable. Whereas calorie intake can be held fairly constant, it can be difficult to maintain constant levels of calorie expenditure. Metabolic factors differ from person to person, and the amount of water retained by the body can vary from day to day. Therefore it is not unusual for someone on a calorie-restricted diet to lose weight in a highly irregular fashion, sometimes remaining on a plateau for weeks at a time. As weight decreases the metabolic rate slows down, as if to defend the body against starvation. Fewer calories are needed by the body, so caloric intake may need to be further decreased, thus creating a cycle that will eventually prove detrimental to the body.

Weight loss can be facilitated by increasing calorie expenditure through exercise. However, it takes a considerable amount of exercise to match the effect of calorie restriction. For example, a vigorous squash game with active play lasting 30 minutes may result in an expenditure of 300 calories. The same net calorie loss could be accomplished just by passing up a single serving of lemon meringue pie. Nevertheless, over the long term, the number of calories burned through regular exercise can total quite a few pounds.

Some people believe that exercise increases appetite, making it even harder to limit eating. Actually, moderate exercise doesn't usually increase appetite and sometimes decreases it. Ideally, a weight-reduction program should result in loss of fat, not muscle. Dieters who don't exercise will lose both. Dieters who do exercise will lose weight mostly as fat. Exercise does not have to be vigorous in order to be effective. Walking at a moderate pace can expend just as many calories as that squash match—it will just take longer.

For many people, walking is ideal exercise because it requires no costly equipment, rarely produces injuries, and can be done as a pleasant social experience. Like other weight-bearing exercises, walking offers an additional benefit for women: by promoting retention of calcium in the bones, it can help prevent osteoporosis. Regular exercise can produce other benefits as well. In addition to increasing muscle tone and stamina, it can reduce the risk of heart disease by improving blood cholesterol levels, reducing high blood pressure, and improving blood sugar levels in diabetics.

Modification of eating habits is essential to a weight-control program. This involves identifying what environmental and personal factors influence the amount of food you eat and finding ways to avoid or control those influences. In some cases it may be necessary to modify the underlying psychological reasons for overeating. Guidance from a professional or self-help group may be worthwhile and may also provide emotional support.

The Bottom Line

Unfortunately, there is no shortcut to weight reduction or weight control. As hard as losing weight may be, keeping it off is even harder. Long-term control, even with careful medical supervision, has been achieved by only a minority of obese individuals. In most cases, when crash dieting is involved, weight loss is maintained for no more than several months at a time. And the all-too-common "yo-yo" cycle of weight loss followed by weight gain leaves many people worse off than before they started. Some studies even suggest that yo-yoing can cause some of the health problems blamed on obesity, and that weight and the percentage of body fat can increase with successive yo-yo cycles.

Medical consultants for CU believe, somewhat facetiously, that the word "diet" should be stricken from the obesity literature. To be "on a diet" implies that someday one will be "off the diet." The best results for the least cost to health and pocketbook can be obtained by gradual, long-term calorie restriction, regular and well-balanced meals, and moderate exercise. People who really want to lose weight should forget about gimmicks, gadgets, and "going on a diet." For permanent results, they must change their eating and living habits—permanently.

10

The Mercury-Amalgam Scare

"Just how concerned should I be?" the CU reporter asked. Dr. Joel Berger, a dentist in Queens, New York, paused a moment before answering. *"If I were you,"* he said, *"and I had that test at eight o'clock this morning, I'd have called two of my friends and made sure I had those fillings out by nine o'clock tonight."*

Dr. Berger has been an outspoken proponent of the notion that mercury-amalgam fillings are poisoning the populace—a notion reportedly espoused by hundreds of dentists across the country. He has issued his warning on numerous New York City–area radio and television talk shows and has been featured on the "CBS Evening News," where he was shown measuring the mercury level in a patient's mouth. The CU reporter, without revealing his affiliation, had gone to Dr. Berger for a consultation in 1985. Dr. Berger's advice to him was similar to what has been told to thousands of consumers by dentists who remove allegedly dangerous fillings and replace them with new ones.

One hundred million Americans have "silver" fillings. The fillings are actually alloys, or amalgams, of silver and several other metals. One of those metals is mercury, which makes up about half the filling. After the puttylike amalgam is inserted, it hardens completely in about one day.

Until recently, scientists believed that the amalgam released mercury vapor only while it was hardening. But in 1979 University of Iowa researchers found that chewing can release minute amounts of mercury vapor from old fillings. That finding sparked the present controversy over amalgam safety.

It's been known for centuries that mercury is a potent poison when swallowed, inhaled, or absorbed through the skin. Exposure to high levels for a long time can damage the brain and nervous system. The classic example occurred during the nineteenth century, when makers of felt hats dipped material into mercuric-nitrate solution to make the felt easier to shape. In so doing, the workers absorbed mercury through their skin and inhaled mercury vapor. Tremors, incoherent speech, difficulty in walking, and feeblemindedness resulted. The problem was immortalized in the phrase "mad as a hatter" and by the Mad Hatter in *Alice in Wonderland*.

Exposure to smaller amounts of mercury vapor can cause less drastic symptoms, including insomnia, anxiety, and minor tremors. Even today, mercury is a hazard for some workers— mainly those in thermometer factories and in plants that use mercury to make chlorine and caustic soda.

Can mercury in fillings cause these or other health problems? That's the key question in the mercury-amalgam controversy. "Antiamalgam" dentists such as Dr. Berger contend that mercury fumes from amalgams can cause problems ranging from depression and multiple sclerosis to fatigue and irritability. Their solution: drill out the amalgams and replace them with fillings made from other materials.

The American Dental Association (ADA), on the other hand, insists that amalgam fillings are safe. Only people allergic to mercury—probably less than 1 percent of the population—need avoid them, the ADA says. And that number is minuscule. According to a special report in the April 1990 *Journal of the American Dental Association*, although billions of amalgam fillings have been used successfully, fewer than fifty cases of allergy have been reported in the scientific literature since 1905.

Dentists don't make up amalgam containing mercury out of any special love for the stuff. They use it because it's strong and durable. Chewing exerts tremendous force on the back teeth—mouthful after mouthful, meal after meal, day after day. An amalgam filling can withstand that force for a long time before breaking down. Mercury-amalgam fillings usually last five to 10 years, and some of them last as long as 40 years.

The main alternatives to mercury-amalgam fillings are composite resin fillings, which were introduced in the 1960s and are made mainly of plastics. When amalgam fillings are removed because of "mercury toxicity," composite fillings usually take their place.

Composites can be mixed to match the color of the tooth and so are often used for front teeth, where cosmetic considerations are important. But composites have several drawbacks, particularly in back teeth, where they are subjected to heavy biting pressure. Typically, they have lasted no more than three years. They're also more expensive than amalgam; and teeth filled with composites are less resistant to recurrent decay.

Composites are being continually tested and improved. Research is under way on composites that can be chemically bonded to teeth. Dental consultants for CU say that composites strong enough for use in back teeth may become available sometime in the 1990s.

Gold inlays may also be used instead of amalgams. They're durable but cost a lot, both for the gold and for the installation, because they must be preshaped to fit the cavity and then cemented into place. They're not a very practical alternative to amalgam fillings.

When the reporter had called Dr. Berger's office for a consultation in 1985, the secretary had asked, "What are your problems?" It was the Monday after a rough weekend. "Fatigue and headaches," the reporter answered. She told him he needed to come in for the mercury toxicity test.

So there he was, with a rubber tube in his mouth. Dr. Berger held the tube there for about 10 seconds as it sucked a small amount of air into a mercury-vapor analyzer. The first measurement was reassuring. The digital readout said zero. Then Dr. Berger told the reporter to chew a stick of gum vigorously for 10 minutes. The measurement taken afterward was 32—which prompted Dr. Berger's "out by nine o'clock tonight" recommendation.

Dr. Berger said that 32 meant a mercury-vapor level of 32 micrograms per cubic meter. Government regulations, he explained, require that workers cannot be exposed to an average mercury-vapor level of more than 50 micrograms per cubic meter of air during an eight-hour working day.

A worker exposed to the CU reporter's mercury level, Dr. Berger said, would be regarded as having a "borderline toxic" exposure. And he would be carefully monitored for five years for signs of mercury poisoning.

A saliva test produced more bad news. According to Dr. Berger, the reporter's "highly acidic" saliva was corroding his fillings and adding to the mercury vapor released during chewing.

The message was clear: the reporter's fillings were endangering his health. How much would it cost to take them out and put nonmercury

*ones in? Dr. Berger counted the number of fillings—eight—and gave
his answer: $580.*

*"Will removal of my fillings cure my fatigue and headaches?" the
reporter asked. Dr. Berger said he couldn't promise that, since it
would depend on the reporter's "unique physiological response" to
mercury. But he said that many of his patients with the same problems
had experienced relief once their fillings were out.*

The mercury-vapor analyzer is a device customarily used
in factories, where it measures the mercury levels in the air.
Is it appropriate for dentists to use it, as some of them are
doing?

The CU dental consultants say that use of the mercury
analyzer is a scare tactic to get patients to part with their
fillings. The consultants say that the device makes it easy for
a dentist to contend that mercury doses exceed occupational
standards.

When using the analyzer, the dentist has the patient chew
vigorously for 10 minutes, creating heat and friction that max-
imize the release of mercury vapor. The analyzer senses the
mercury contained in about half a cup of air and multiplies it
by 8,000. That gives a readout corresponding to the mercury
level in a cubic meter of air—about the amount inhaled in an
hour. But for the patient, the exposure doesn't last for hours.
It lasts only a few minutes during chewing—and only a frac-
tion of the vapor may be inhaled. Most people don't inhale
through their mouth when chewing. And even when they're
not chewing, most people breathe through the nose, so that
inhaled air bypasses any mercury vapor that may be in their
mouth. One recent study showed that the analyzer technique
tends to produce estimates that are some 16 times higher than
the actual daily dose of mercury vapor.

In assessing mercury vapor's effect on health, the key question is: how much actually gets absorbed by the body's tissues?

Dr. Thomas W. Clarkson of the University of Rochester School of Medicine is one of the world's leading authorities on mercury toxicity. He says that a mercury-vapor analyzer can't answer that question. Clarkson told CU that mercury exposure can best be assessed by measuring the mercury levels in blood and urine. The urine level provides the best measure of "body burden," or long-term exposure to mercury, whereas the blood level reflects recent exposure.

"I can promise one thing," Dr. Berger said. "Removal of your fillings will definitely lower your body burden of mercury."

The reporter wondered: just how heavy was his body's mercury burden? After all, he'd presumably been gulping mercury vapor ever since his first filling at age nine. And corrosive saliva had presumably been his constant companion. Two hours after leaving Dr. Berger's office, he was in the office of CU's chief medical consultant, where he had his saliva tested for acidity and provided a blood sample and a urine specimen.

In those two hours, his saliva had changed from "highly acidic" to neutral. The blood and urine samples were analyzed for mercury by a leading biomedical laboratory. The blood level was well within the normal range. For urine, the level was six micrograms per liter. Normal, according to the lab, is anything up to 20 micrograms per liter.

The reporter notified Dr. Clarkson of his test results. Dr. Clarkson's advice: "Hold on to your $580."

Almost everyone, Dr. Clarkson said, has detectable levels of mercury in the urine and blood. The main source of mercury in most people's bodies is the food they eat, seafood in particular. Dr. Clarkson expressed surprise that the CU reporter, who eats tuna at lunch most days, had such modest mercury levels in his blood and urine.

If dental amalgams really were poisoning people, Dr. Clarkson pointed out, the mercury levels in the general population (where fillings are commonplace) would rival those found among workers exposed to mercury. That's far from the case. In one study of 1,107 people (mainly in the United States), 95 percent had urine levels of mercury lower than 20 micrograms. Adverse health effects appear when the level reaches about 150 micrograms or more, Dr. Clarkson said.

The CU dental consultants point out that replacing mercury fillings may cost more than money. Reinvading a tooth—drilling out amalgam and installing a replacement—can increase tooth sensitivity and weaken the tooth. In addition, studies show that drilling out amalgam can produce brief but significant increases in mercury levels in the mouth.

In one case—which sparked a lawsuit—a California woman charged that a dentist had fraudulently removed five amalgam fillings after telling her that they were a "liability" to her large intestine. The woman subsequently suffered pulpal irritation which required extraction of two teeth and root canal therapy in two others. The suit was settled for $100,000 in 1985.

If anyone faces a health hazard from mercury fillings, it's dentists and their assistants. The average dentist handles between two and three pounds of mercury every year. Skin contact can result in absorption. Careless use and accidental spills can produce significant levels of mercury vapor in the air. Surveys have shown that as many as 10 percent of dental offices have mercury-vapor levels about 50 micrograms per cubic meter of air—the upper limit that the National Institute for Occupational Safety and Health considers safe for eight-hour exposures in the workplace. But despite their higher exposure, dental personnel aren't being poisoned. Since 1982 the ADA has sponsored a mercury testing service that measures urine-mercury levels in dentists and others who work in dental offices. Although average levels are about four times higher than in the general population, they are still well within the acceptable range.

According to CU's dental consultants, a major reason some dentists are riding the antiamalgam bandwagon can be summed up in one word: fluoride. Largely because of fluoridated drinking water and fluoride toothpastes, the incidence of tooth decay over the past two decades has been cut roughly in half. So some dentists are suffering from a large cavity in their practice. Taking out and replacing amalgam fillings helps fill their financial hole.

Leading Antiamalgamists

Have you felt draggy, listless and even fatigued when you wake up? Have you felt depressed, irritable and jumpy, and lashed out at people for no good reason? Have you worried yourself sick because thoughts of suicide keep floating into your conscious mind? For many of my patients, the culprit is mercury toxicity.

So writes Dr. Hal Huggins, spiritual leader of the antiamalgam movement. Dr. Huggins, whose activities are centered in Colorado Springs, claims that at least 20 percent of people with amalgam fillings are "mercury toxic"—and that the ADA "is covering up the fact" because of its fear of lawsuits.

Dr. Huggins gets his message out through books, articles, tapes, and lectures. In 1985 he told CU that he had spoken to between 4,000 and 5,000 dentists, 1,500 of whom had attended his seminars on mercury toxicity. Each day, he said, his office fielded about 250 letters and phone calls from concerned members of the public.

Dr. Huggins said that he hadn't practiced dentistry for two and a half years. Instead, he was involved in "diagnosis and treatment planning." A three-to-four-hour consultation with Huggins cost about $1,500. Or for $300, patients could get a consultation through the mail after completing a computerized questionnaire and submitting hair and urine samples for analysis.

Dr. Huggins reported that he had treated about 150 patients with multiple sclerosis and that 80 percent of them had experienced "substantial improvement." In 1983 such claims prompted the National Multiple Sclerosis Society to issue a memo to all its chapters. In it, the society said that no evidence existed that multiple sclerosis was related to dental amalgams, and that "this therapeutic claim . . . involves economic implications, in terms of expense to the patient and great profit to the dentist."

In 1989 the ADA Council on Ethics, Bylaws and Judicial Affairs concluded that any dentist who represents dental treatment as a cure for disease, infection, or other condition, without the support of accepted scientific knowledge or research, is acting unethically. The ruling was triggered in part by the case of an Iowa dentist whose license was suspended for extracting all 28 of a patient's teeth supposedly because doing so might relieve or arrest the progress of multiple sclerosis. The dentist's license was suspended for nine months, and he was placed on probation for an additional four years and three months.

"The suicidal patient," Dr. Huggins has written, "is very special to us." He told CU that his success with suicidal patients had been "better than 50 percent." For some of these depressed people, he said, "it just takes a couple of weeks and it's gone." He also claimed that mercury toxicity causes many other conditions, including epilepsy, leukemia, Hodgkin's disease, arthritis, mononucleosis, and premenstrual syndrome.

Dr. Huggins described his approach in his 1985 book, *It's All in Your Head*—which prompted the Colorado attorney general's office to investigate whether he was practicing medicine without a license.

Not surprisingly, Dr. Huggins recommends amalgam removal as part of the treatment process. But fillings, he says, must be removed in the proper sequence. That's where the Amalgameter, a Huggins invention, comes in.

This device supposedly reads the "electrical current" in each filling and determines whether the current is "positive" or "negative." Dr. Huggins claims that highly negative fillings (which supposedly cause the worst diseases) must be removed first; otherwise, amalgam removal probably won't help the patient.

Dr. Huggins formed Tox Supply, Incorporated, to market the Amalgameter (cost: $350) to other dentists. In 1985 the FDA informed Dr. Huggins that the Amalgameter's promotion and distribution involved "serious violations of the Federal Food, Drug and Cosmetic Act." The FDA said that "there is no scientific basis for the removal of dental amalgams for the purposes claimed." By that time, Dr. Huggins had sold Tox Supply, Incorporated, but, according to the FDA, he continued to recommend the Amalgameter's use.

When people are "mercury toxic," amalgam's removal is not enough, according to Dr. Huggins. He also recommends special nutritional supplements "to get rid of the body's stored mercury." Dr. Huggins markets the supplements through his company, Matrix Minerals, Incorporated. Two of them, *X-IT* and *Eater's Digest*, prompted a warning from the FDA in 1985. The FDA charged that both products were "unapproved new drugs" whose labeling was false and misleading.

Dr. Huggins claims to have been studying mercury toxicity since 1973. But when CU asked him for evidence in 1985 that amalgam fillings can harm people, he acknowledged that he had no clinical studies. His evidence, he said, was contained in the 600 case studies stored in his computer. They have provided "a massive amount" of data that "all points in the same direction." Dr. Huggins told CU, "As soon as I take my course in statistics, I will start putting together the information." During the past year, according to his published literature, Dr. Huggins has been promoting *Jogger Juice,* a vitamin/mineral "energy drink" he claims is effective in combating fatigue, increasing alertness, and lowering blood pressure.

In addition to Hal Huggins and Joel Berger, some prominent antiamalgamists include:

• *Michael F. Ziff,* an Orlando, Florida, dentist who, in 1985, was traveling around the country giving courses to dentists on mercury toxicity. He claims to have "completed research on over 400 articles on mercury toxicity." Ziff boasts a "B.S. degree in nutrition" from Donsbach University, an unaccredited school that taught a broad range of unscientific concepts.

• *Sam Ziff,* Michael Ziff's father, is the author of the book *Silver Dental Fillings: The Toxic Time Bomb.* He and his son Michael have written a booklet, "The Hazards of Silver Mercury Dental Fillings," which antiamalgam dentists give away to their patients. Sam Ziff also has a degree from Donsbach University—in his case, a "Ph.D."

• *Roy Kupsinel*, M.D., of Oviedo, Florida, publishes *Health Consciousness*—a "holistic" magazine that carries numerous articles opposing mercury-amalgam fillings. He has marketed Amalgameters and has written a booklet called "A Patient's Guide to Mercury Amalgam Toxicity." He also founded and is vice president of the American Quack Association. In a 1987 article in *Health Consciousness*, he said he had once suffered from mercury-amalgam toxicity; hypoglycemia; allergies to foods, chemicals, and inhalants; chronic candidiasis; hypothyroidism; and several other "common denominators of degenerative disease." He also described how he was expelled from his county and state medical societies during the mid-1970s after complaints were made to the county society about his "nutritional/hypoglycemia practice."

Conclusions

Amalgams have been used for more than 150 years. Except for a few people with a genuine allergy to mercury, CU knows of no reliable studies that show anyone has been harmed by them. There's little danger of the United States becoming a nation of Mad Hatters.

In CU's view, dentists who purport to treat health problems by ripping out fillings are putting their own economic interests ahead of their patients' welfare. The false diagnosis of mercury-amalgam toxicity has such harmful potential and shows such poor judgment on the part of the practitioner that CU believes dentists who engage in this practice should have their licenses revoked.

At least one state licensing agency seems to share this viewpoint. In March 1990, the New York State Board of Dental

Examiners revoked Joel Berger's license after he was charged with inappropriately removing a patient's amalgam fillings as a treatment for arm and leg pain. The board concluded that Dr. Berger's testing procedures (the same that CU's reporter had undergone) were beyond the scope of dental practice and "had no basis in scientific fact."

11

Chiropractic:
Still Not Recommended

Chiropractors are licensed to practice in all fifty states. Their schools, most of which are accredited, award a Doctor of Chiropractic (D.C.) degree. Their services are partially included under Medicare and are covered in most states by private insurance carriers, Blue Shield plans, worker's compensation plans, and Medicaid. More than 40,000 chiropractors are now practicing, and many have achieved a large following of satisfied patients. But the nature and quality of what chiropractors do can vary greatly from practitioner to practitioner, and much of what they do is unscientific or unethical.

Humble Beginnings

Chiropractic, which literally means "done by hand," was the brainchild of Daniel David Palmer, a tradesman who operated a "magnetic healing" studio in Davenport, Iowa, late in the nineteenth century. One of Palmer's passions had been to discover the ultimate cause of disease—why one person should be ill while another person, "eating at the same table, working in the same shop," was spared illness. Today we know that heredity and the body's immune system, among other things, can often make the difference. But according to Palmer, this question was answered in September 1895.

The answer occurred to him, wrote Palmer, after treating a janitor who was so deaf he could not hear the racket of a wagon on the street or the ticking of a watch. Palmer alleged that he restored the man's hearing by pressing on a vertebra (a bony segment of the man's spine). Apparently unaware that the nerves of hearing are located entirely within the skull, Palmer imagined that he had relieved pressure on a spinal nerve that affected hearing. Adjusting the bony segment, he decided, had removed interference with the nerve supply and thereby allowed the body's "Innate Intelligence" to effect a cure. Innate Intelligence, said Palmer, was the "Soul, Spirit or Spark of Life," which expressed itself through the nervous system to control the healing process. By impeding that expression, Palmer concluded, misaligned vertebrae were the cause of most disease.

In 1895 medical science was still in its infancy. Louis Pasteur had only recently demonstrated the plausibility of the germ theory of disease. And little more than a generation separated Palmer from many eminent physicians who had earlier considered the spine to be the seat of innumerable human ills. It had been a common practice, in fact, to apply leeches, irritants, or even hot irons to tender sites along the spine as a treatment for various disorders. By the end of the nineteenth century, however, such practices had waned. The scientific revolution that would extend the boundaries of medicine in the twentieth century had already begun.

Osteopathy, which emerged a few years before chiropractic, adapted to the change. While retaining a separate identity—in part because it used manipulative therapy and emphasized the muscles and skeletal system—osteopathy gradually adopted the concepts and practices of orthodox medical science as well. Osteopathic students now receive training similar to that of medical students and earn a Doctor of Osteopathy (D.O.) degree that enables them to practice on an equal legal footing with medical doctors.

In contrast, chiropractors are still fixated on the spine. Chiropractic's basic problem is not its use of spinal manipulation—a legitimate procedure when done properly—but its theoretical basis for doing so.

"Modern" Theory

Many chiropractors still cling to Palmer's notion that spinal misalignments—which they commonly refer to as "subluxations"—are the principal cause of disease. According to a 1980 pamphlet from the Parker Chiropractic Research Foundation, for example, subluxation is "a disease occurring worldwide in epidemic proportions . . . as much as 90 percent of the world's population suffers from subluxation of varying degree interfering with the function of the body and, therefore, with normal health." Some chiropractors have even advertised that vertebral subluxations kill millions of people yearly.

On the other hand, "modern" chiropractic has modified Palmer's theories to accommodate some basic scientific realities. Modern chiropractic, for example, agrees with medicine that germs are factors in disease and that the body has inherent defense mechanisms against them. However, it still claims that mechanical disturbances of the nervous system impair the body's defenses and are an underlying cause of disease. According to this theory, minor "off-centerings" or "fixations" of the vertebrae can disturb nerve function, lower the body's resistance to germs, and cause or aggravate disease by disturbing nerve impulses to the visceral organs. Some chiropractors maintain that chiropractic deals with the cause of disease, whereas medicine merely deals with the symptoms.

The American Chiropractic Association (ACA), which is the nation's largest chiropractic organization, has said for years that "while many factors impair man's health, disturbances of the nervous system are among the most important." A 1980 survey of 1,000 chiropractors selected from the ACA's mailing list found that only 37 (14 percent) of 268 respondents did not believe that the chiropractic subluxation is a significant cause of disease. In a 1988 ad in the *Reader's Digest*, the ACA said that "functional disorders, such as those that involve organs and glands, may respond to chiropractic adjustments." And in the November 1989 *ACA Journal of Chiropractic*, a recent graduate of New York Chiropractic College urged his colleagues to "always keep our sights focused on the primary objective of reducing subluxations to benefit all."

According to Louis Sportelli, D.C., a recent chairman of the ACA's board of governors, "regular spinal adjustments are a part of your body's defense against illness." His booklet "Introduction to Chiropractic"—more than two million copies of which have been purchased by chiropractors for distribution to the public—says, "If parents were as concerned about having their children's spines checked for minor derangements (subluxations) as they are about having their teeth checked for cavities, they would be helping their youngsters attain a healthier state of well-being. Proper spinal care is essential to your child's health."

Treatment Methods

Although basic chiropractic theory has been modified somewhat since 1895, the primary treatment is still the spinal "adjustment"—or manipulation. Most chiropractors do this by hand, pressing on the back, though some use a mechanical device. The choice of vertebrae to adjust and the degree of force to exert vary with the philosophy of the practitioner. Some chiropractors believe that only the topmost spinal bones need adjusting; some hold that the lowermost (sacral) bones are the key to health; some focus on both ends; and others relate specific levels to specific organs or diseases. Some chiropractors use very slight pressure, whereas others are far more vigorous. When manipulation is done quickly, it often produces a "click" in the manipulated joint, similar to the popping of a knuckle.

Osteopaths, physical therapists, athletic trainers, and some medical doctors—specialists in physical medicine—also use manipulative techniques for certain musculoskeletal problems. Stephen M. Levin, M.D., a former president of the North American Academy of Manipulative Medicine (now called the North American Academy of Musculoskeletal Medicine), estimates that about 8,000 physicians worldwide use manipulative techniques. The prevailing scientific viewpoint, says Dr. Levin, an orthopedist in Alexandria, Virginia, who limits his practice to the treatment of back pain, is that manipulation relieves pain and secondary muscle spasm by restoring the mobility of joints that have a mechanical malfunction. "When I meet with scientifically oriented chiropractors, including educators at some of their better schools, we talk the same language," says Dr. Levin. "In fact, some of them say that patients who aren't better within two weeks should be referred elsewhere."

Although some of their academic leaders may be aligned with the scientific community, most practicing chiropractors still tell their patients that manipulation is done to correct "subluxations." The chiropractor "subluxation" is so loosely defined, however, that it takes in virtually any mechanical or functional derangement of the spine—or, as one observer has put it, "any variance from the normalcy of a newborn child."

Despite chiropractic's origin and all-embracing theory of disease, the public tends to view chiropractors as specialists in muscle or joint problems, particularly those of the back. Part of the reason, or course, is that chiropractic manipulation focuses on the spine. Whatever its ultimate intent, the therapy involves direct, physical action on the back. So people may conclude that that's what the treatment is for.

But there are other reasons for this traditional association. For one thing, the medical doctor in the early days of chiropractic gave little priority to back ailments. The new science of bacteriology held immense promise for treating otherwise fatal illnesses, as did other developments in diagnosis and in surgery. Hence medical efforts in the first third of this century focused on infectious disease and similarly urgent problems. Backaches could wait. Not until the 1930s did the medical profession start paying much attention to physical medicine and rehabilitation. In the interim, chiropractic seemed to offer hope in an area that medicine had largely ignored.

Even today, many physicians find little satisfaction in treating back ailments. Chronic pain may often be influenced by psychological problems or by physical habits that patients are unable or unwilling to change. Exact diagnosis can be elusive and expensive, and follow-up treatment can be time-consuming for the doctor. Specialists in physical medicine and orthopedics interviewed by CU asserted that, too often, treatment by some physicians simply has meant prescribing a painkiller, muscle relaxant, or tranquilizer rather than taking the time and effort that such ailments might demand.

Chiropractors, meanwhile, have usually been ready and willing to see patients repeatedly and to provide active treatment—manipulation, exercise programs, heat application, and the like. In CU's opinion, such accommodation has probably reinforced the belief the chiropractors specialize in back ailments.

Chiropractors who belong to the International Chiropractors Association tend to confine their treatment to manipulation. Besides spinal adjustment, treatment may include various "soft-tissue" manipulations, such as massaging muscles or applying sustained pressure to ligaments. But the basic approach is "hands only."

The majority of chiropractors, however, use a variety of treatment techniques. The scope of their practice generally depends on what's permitted by state law. Chiropractors do not perform surgery or prescribe medications. But many jurisdictions allow them to use physical therapy and to recommend various nutritional supplements, such as vitamins and minerals. Some chiropractors' treatments are identical or similar to some used by physicians or physical therapists—although the stated purpose may not be the same. In addition to exercise programs, such measures may include the use of a brace or cast, whirlpool baths, hot or cold packs, ultrasound, diathermy (deep heat treatments), and other devices. Some chiropractors also use megavitamins, "glandulars," herbal products, reflexology, acupuncture, acupressure, colonics, iridology, and other dubious approaches described in Appendix 2.

The range of dubious chiropractic care has been revealed by three large studies in which investigators consulted multiple chiropractors for checkups:

• During the 1970s the Lehigh Valley Committee Against Health Fraud sent three healthy volunteers to a total of 16 chiropractors in or near Allentown, Pennsylvania. Fifteen of the chiropractors recommended treatment, but no two agreed on where the supposed problems were located. Committee representatives also asked 35 local chiropractors how often people who feel well should have their spine checked. The majority of answers ranged from four to 12 times a year.

• In 1981 Mark Brown, a reporter for the *Quad-City Times*, a newspaper in Davenport, Iowa, conducted a five-month investigation of chiropractors during which he visited about two dozen of them as a "patient." He reported that each one said he was a "chiropractic case," and that all but one insisted on X rays before treatment. One chiropractor placed a potato and an egg on the reporter's chest to test the strength of his arms, held a magnet over his thymus gland, concluded that nutrient deficiencies were present, and sold him four bottles of "glandular" substances for $47.50. Another chiropractor passed a cylindrical instrument over the reporter's back and marked any spots over which the instrument made a squeaking noise. Another claimed to diagnose subluxations by using an instrument that recorded temperature differences from one side of the spine to another. Another examined the reporter's eyes for markings that would indicate what diseases were found within the body. Another told the reporter his ears were acting as "antennae for nerve energy" that had become congested in his diaphragm. Brown also reported that on one day during his investigation, one chiropractor informed him his left leg was shorter than his right and another chiropractor told him just the opposite. Other chiropractors also said that he suffered from hiatal hernia, "ileocecal valve syndrome," and "ocular lock."

• During 1989 William M. London, Ed.D., assistant professor of health education at Kent State University, visited 23 chiropractors in Ohio and Florida who had advertised free consultations or examinations. Every one of them espoused subluxation theory either during the consultation or in waiting room literature, and all but two recommended periodic preventive maintenance. Seventeen performed examinations. Of these, three identified subluxations (at differing locations), three said his left leg was shorter than his right leg, and two said his right leg was shorter than his left. Seven recommended treatment.

Despite such goings-on, chiropractic leaders have long insisted that chiropractors should be considered primary physicians. They claim chiropractors are qualified to be "portals of entry" to the health-care system, functioning essentially as family doctors and referring patients, when appropriate, to other health professionals. Some chiropractors even suggest that when illness occurs, a person should "try chiropractic first, medicine second, and surgery last." This assumes that chiropractors will recognize when to treat a patient and when to refer one to a physician—which raises the issue of how chiropractors are trained.

Chiropractic Education

There is virtually no denial that educational standards for chiropractors in the not-so-distant past were appalling. In 1964 Dewey Anderson, Ph.D., then director of education for the ACA, reported the results of a comprehensive evaluation of chiropractic schools: "Too many instructors teaching the basic sciences without having had any advanced or graduate training in these sciences. Too many instructors not trained or qualified as teachers nor masters of their fields, resulting in slavish devotion to textbook teaching and instruction considerably below the level of post-college professional education." Anderson also noted that students were similarly unqualified: "One of the most serious handicaps . . . is that of trying to teach at the post-college professional level students who for the most part have not gone beyond high school, and who in high school were not in the upper half of their classes. For many of them a professional college course is too difficult to master." The result, said Anderson, was to downgrade instruction so that students could pass the courses.

Landmark studies of chiropractic by the U.S. Department of Health, Education, and Welfare (now Department of Health and Human Services) in 1968 and Ontario's Committee on the Healing Arts in 1970 expressed similarly critical findings. In addition to poorly qualified teachers, inferior basic science courses, and notably low admission requirements, both reports criticized the paucity of research. The HEW report also noted the absence of inpatient hospital training and a poor ratio of faculty to students. At the time of the HEW study, chiropractic schools averaged about one faculty member for each 19 students, compared with one per 1.7 students in medical schools. (Both sets of figures included part-time instructors with administrative duties or outside practices.) The report concluded: "Chiropractic theory and practice are not based upon the body of basic knowledge related to health, disease, and health care that has been widely accepted by the scientific community. Moreover, irrespective of its theory, the scope and quality of chiropractic education do not prepare the practitioner to make an adequate diagnosis and provide appropriate treatment." The Ontario committee endorsed the HEW findings on education and judged the chiropractor's diagnostic ability as very limited at best.

Since that time, chiropractic schools have raised their educational standards considerably. They still require only a "C" average for admission, but entering students must have at least two years of college work, including courses in biology, chemistry, and physics. (Actually, the overall grade-point average of entering students has been a "B," and about half have a college degree.) Academic requirements for faculty members have also been upgraded, so that instructors in basic-science subjects now have recognized credentials in the fields in which they teach.

Despite improvements in other areas, chiropractic education in diagnosis remains inferior to the training received by physicians. In the practice of medicine, differential diagnosis—that is, one that considers possible causes of a patient's symptoms and establishes probable as well as alternative diagnoses—is fundamental. But chiropractors traditionally believed it wasn't important to "name" a disease. The important thing was to find and correct the subluxation allegedly causing it. It made little difference if, say, a liver disorder involved congestion, cirrhosis, or cancer; the object was to relieve nervous-system disturbances that were supposedly responsible for the disorder. Chiropractors preferred to call their approach "spinal analysis" rather than diagnosis. Even today, some practitioners insist that medical diagnosis is out of place in chiropractic.

Most chiropractic association officials and educators disagree with that sentiment. Diagnostic training is part of the curriculum at chiropractic colleges, and some colleges even have physicians teaching it. But the instructional programs still do not provide sufficient clinical experience in diagnosing and treating the gamut of problems faced by practicing physicians. The range of ailments seen in patients attending clinics at chiropractic schools is far narrower than that of patients seen at medical school clinics, and chiropractic students have little or no hospital training. In addition, chiropractors are not trained or permitted to use many of the sophisticated diagnostic techniques available to physicians, including some major diagnostic aids involving the spine.

Nor do chiropractors have the benefit of the more extensive education and training required of physicians. In contrast to the chiropractors' two years of college and four years of professional school, medical and osteopathic physicians must have four years of college, four years of medical school, and usually three or more years of hospital residency training. Moreover, university and community hospitals throughout the United States are centers where medical knowledge is reinforced and expanded through conferences, discussions, and association with colleagues, as well as through experiences with patients. The scope of educational programs sponsored by chiropractic colleges and professional organizations is limited.

More fundamental than the quality of the educational process, however, is the validity of what chiropractors are taught. As one prominent critic has remarked, "Can a house be built without a foundation?"

Chiropractic and Science

The belief that minor interference with spinal nerves can cause or aggravate disease is still the cornerstone of chiropractic theory. It is also the focus of scientific objections. A few anatomical facts may help explain why. Twenty-six pairs of nerves exit from mobile segments of the spine. They are the only part of the nervous system conceivably accessible to manipulation. Twelve pairs of cranial nerves, which exit through openings in the base of the skull and bypass the spine, are out of reach of manipulation. So, too, are five pairs exiting from the sacrum, a solid bone formed by the fusion of five vertebrae in the lower spine. The spinal cord (which is surrounded by protective layers of tissue) and the brain itself—with all its interconnecting nerve pathways—are also out of reach.

Thus the chiropractor's action addresses only a part of the nervous system. It excludes, for example, the nerves of sight, hearing, taste, and smell, and the entire parasympathetic nervous system. The latter, along with the sympathetic nervous system, form the balancing halves of the autonomic (involuntary) nervous system, which serves the vital organs.

Scientists, of course, accept the importance of the nervous system in body functions. But they reject any assertion that manipulation directed at a limited part of this intricate system can prevent or cure disease. In the first place, there's no scientific evidence that minor "off-centerings" of the vertebrae impinge on spinal nerves. In fact, Edmund Crelin, Ph.D., a prominent anatomist at Yale University, has proved that it cannot happen. In a study published in 1973 in *American Scientist*, he demonstrated with cadavers that impingement cannot occur even when the spine is twisted unless the force applied is so great that it would disable or kill a living person. Second, if minor spinal nerve pressure could occur, its effect would be nil. Research by neurophysiologists shows that a nerve impulse travels more slowly in a zone of partial compression but resumes its flow immediately thereafter. The impulse transmitted is normal in all respects.

Chiropractors also have their own concept of the nervous system as a whole. According to that view, the nervous system is the master of all body functions, regulating everything from major organs to intricate cellular activities. A typical statement of this concept appears in "How Chiropractic Heals," a pamphlet for patients circulated in the 1970s. According to this pamphlet, "None of the body functions 'just happen.' Your heart doesn't just happen to beat. Your lungs don't just happen to inhale and exhale. Your stomach doesn't just happen to digest your dinner. All doctors know that your brain and nerve system coordinate these functions which make for life instead of death, health instead of sickness."

Actually, all doctors—at least doctors of medicine—know no such thing. The heart *does* just happen to beat. It will beat for a period of time even if removed from the body and cut off from all nerve impulses, so long as it's surrounded by a nutrient fluid. Transplanted, it is capable of sustaining life in another human being without any direct connection to the brain, spinal cord, or other nerve tissue. The heart has an intrinsic rhythm of its own and thus can function automatically.

Inherent processes govern the functions of organs as important as the heart, stomach, intestines, blood vessels, and the like. Their function doesn't depend entirely on the nervous system. A paraplegic woman may conceive, carry her pregnancy to term, and give birth to a normal baby—despite severe injury to her spinal cord. Except for bladder and bowel problems, internal organs of quadriplegics still continue to function, even though connections between the brain and many of the body's vital organs have been severed. In short, life can go on despite even massive "interference" with nerve impulses. That doesn't mean the spinal nerves aren't important. But their importance doesn't render other fundamental life processes trivial.

The immunological defense system can also work independently of nerve impulses. Artificially cultured white blood cells will continue to engulf germs even though entirely divorced from nerve influence. At the cellular level, to which chiropractic often claims to extend, the same autonomy has been documented. These biochemical life processes are fundamental—and completely independent of the nervous system. No scientific study has ever shown that manipulation can affect any of these processes, but a vast amount of evidence suggests it cannot.

In 1895 neither Palmer nor his contemporaries could foresee that research. Today, however, there's no excuse for ignoring it. Unless most medical research in the twentieth century is wrong, Palmer's disease theory belongs in the pages of nineteenth-century history, along with bleeding, purging, and other blind alleys of medicine.

The Elusive "Subluxation"

About 30 years ago, when the National Association of Letter Carriers included chiropractic in its insurance plan, it received claims for chiropractic treatment of cancer, heart disease, mumps, mental retardation, and many other questionable conditions. When asked to justify such claims by sending X-ray evidence of spinal problems, chiropractors submitted hundreds of X-ray films that supposedly contained subluxations. However, when chiropractic association officials were asked to review the X rays, they were unable to point out a single subluxation.

In 1973, when Congress included chiropractic under Medicare, the law stated that payment would be made for "subluxations demonstrated by X rays to exist." To help chiropractors get paid, the American Chiropractic Association issued four editions of a *Basic Chiropractic Procedural Manual*, which define subluxations as anything that could interfere with spinal function. "Since we are obligated to find subluxations before receiving payment," the first (1974) manual warned, "it behooves us to make an objective study of what [X-ray] films show in the way of subluxations." Referring to the Letter Carriers experience as an "unfortunate debacle which almost destroyed chiropractic credibility in Washington," the ACA warned: *the subluxations must be perfectly obvious and indisputable.* Obvious or not, chiropractors have continued to collect hundreds of millions of Medicare dollars for treating "subluxations."

In 1986 the U.S. Department of Health and Human Services' Office of the Inspector General (OIG) reported on a telephone survey of 145 chiropractors. While 122 (84 percent) of the respondents told OIG investigators that some subluxations do not show on X rays, nearly half said that when billing Medicare, they "could always find something" (by X ray or physical examination) to justify the diagnosis, or actually tailored the diagnosis to obtain reimbursement. The OIG report concluded that "the x-ray requirement is not currently well enforced, may be unenforceable and is highly conducive to abuse." It also concluded that despite evidence of an increased emphasis on science and professionalism in the training and practice of chiropractors, "there also exist patterns of activity and practice which at best appear as overly aggressive marketing—and, in some cases, seem deliberately aimed at misleading patients and the public regarding chiropractic care."

In 1984 some clear-thinking chiropractors formed the National Association for Chiropractic Medicine with hopes that they could help place chiropractic on a sound, scientific basis. To gain admission to this group, applicants must sign a written pledge to "openly renounce the historical chiropractic philosophical concept that subluxation is the cause of disease," and to restrict their scope of practice to "neuromusculoskeletal conditions of a nonsurgical nature." So far, about 100 chiropractors and chiropractic students have joined.

Practice-Building Techniques

A 1988 survey conducted by the American Chiropractic Association found that its members had a median gross income of $174,500 with a net of $78,500. Chiropractors can boost their income considerably by using techniques taught by "practice-building" organizations that abound within the profession. Some of these charge a modest fee for a few days of instruction, whereas others charge thousands of dollars or a percentage of a chiropractor's increased income above a figure based on the chiropractor's past performance.

The oldest practice-building firm is the Parker Chiropractor Research Foundation, of Fort Worth, Texas. Ads for its Parker School for Professional Success have claimed that more than two-thirds of practicing chiropractors have attended its 300 seminars, that tens of thousands of "extra patients" have been served as a result, and that increased income to chiropractic was "into the billions."

Another seminar held regularly is the Dynamic Essentials program developed by Sid E. Williams, D.C., who has been president of the International Chiropractors Association and founded two of chiropractic's 17 current American colleges. Williams's 254-page *Dynamic Essentials of the Chiropractic Principle, Practice and Procedure*, acquired by CU in the late 1970s, provides detailed instructions on how to persuade all patients to have their spines checked and adjusted once a month for life. On page 218, for example, he advises: "Keep in mind that we don't want to feature 'Well' or 'Cure' too soon or too strongly because the patient won't show up for the next visit. . . . He is never well—just better. Don't emphasize improvement too fast. Instead we say, 'We want to get you over on the good side of the ledger and keep you there.' "

Practice Management Associates (PMA), a Florida-based firm run by Peter Fernandez, D.C., advertises that graduates who follow PMA's guidelines gross an average of $235,000 in their first year of practice and that the average gross income of their clients is about $350,000. Fernandez, who teaches that everyone has subluxations that need adjusting, has written a five-book series called *Secrets of a Practice-Building Consultant*. The first volume, his book *1001 Ways to Attract Patients*, published in 1981, includes the following suggestions on how to build one's reputation when beginning chiropractic practice:

> Never go anywhere without being paged. This affixes your name in people's minds. . . . Whenever you're not busy, tell your receptionist that you are going to a certain supermarket, and . . . to have you paged as if for an emergency. . . . This paging procedure can be used 15 to 20 times a day very successfully. . . .
>
> Your wife and/or receptionist can dial any phone number and say, "Is this Dr. So-and-So's, the chiropractor's office? I hear he is tremendous with treating headaches and I've got a terrible headache." . . . I know a doctor who employed a woman to make these calls eight hours a day. It was her only function on his staff! He built a large-volume practice in a short time using this technique. . . .
>
> Write notes on good chiropractic literature . . . with a red pencil: "John, this man cured my head-

aches. Go to him!" Or "Bob, this is the best doctor
in the whole town! He cured the back problem that
I have had for the past 15 years!" Then take this
literature, with your name and location stamped on
it, and lay it all over town.

The fifth volume in Fernandez' series, published in 1990,
is called *How to Become a Million Dollar Practitioner*.

What Do Chiropractors Really Offer?

Despite chiropractic's rejection of science and the excesses of
some practitioners, chiropractors maintain that they offer an
important health service. And each year more than 10 million
Americans obtain chiropractic treatment. Many of these patients sincerely believe that chiropractors help them. But how
many actually benefit from chiropractic treatment? And what
risks do they face in the process?

Many positive responses to chiropractic treatment undoubt-
edly stem from the self-limiting nature of various illnesses or
from the placebo effect of the "laying on of hands." But some
favorable results can be ascribed directly to manipulation itself. Studies in several countries have judged manipulation to
be a useful technique for certain conditions, such as the loss
of joint mobility. Research in manipulation is still meager,
and controlled clinical studies are few. But chiropractors and
other practitioners who use manipulative therapy agree it can
help some muscle or joint problems.

Treatment of tension headaches by massage, for example,
is well recognized. Those headaches can stem from tense
muscles in the neck, and massage may relieve symptoms.
Some practitioners also report that a stiff joint in the neck

may sometimes cause headache pain that can be treated by manipulation.

In general, back or neck pain that might arise from restricted movement in a spinal joint may respond to manipulation. Such pain is usually localized in the area of the joint. Occasionally, however, the pain is felt in another part of the body, where it may mimic the symptoms of a different disorder. For example, a problem in the spine sometimes produces chest pains that resemble angina pectoris.

"Thus we find a perfectly reasonable basis in fact for the somewhat bizarre stories of miraculous cures by spinal manipulation," said John M. Mennell, M.D., another authority on manipulative therapy. "Amost invariably the basis of these stories is that the patient has been told a diagnosis which he believes and remembers," wrote Mennell in his book *Back Pain* (1960). "If his symptoms are then unrelieved by orthodox treatment, but are later cured by a manipulator, it is not surprising that the patient claims to have been cured of the visceral disease." Many chiropractors and other manipulators share Mennell's view.

In short, a variety of possible reasons explain why patients may experience benefits from chiropractic treatment. There are, however, balancing factors to be considered. In addition to money wasted for unnecessary services, there are the potential hazards of treatment that ignores established scientific knowledge. A health practitioner should always avoid exposing a patient to unnecessary risks. The maxim, as a medical aphorism puts it, is *primum non nocere*: "First of all, do no harm."

The ACA asserts that spinal manipulation is a painless and safe procedure. But both chiropractic and medical literature indicates that manipulation is not hazard-free. The reported adverse effects range from minor sprains and soreness to serious complications and even death. Serious complications included fracture, spinal disk rupture, paraplegia, and stroke. These are rare, but when there is no rational basis for using manipulation, they are inexcusable.

Many surgical procedures and drugs used in medical practice are hazardous. Physicians will therefore weigh such risks against the proven value of treatment so that patients will not be endangered unnecessarily. While an individual physician's judgment may be faulty, the emphasis of medicine on *proven* therapy tends to increase a patient's chances of genuine therapeutic benefits for the risks taken.

If spinal manipulation were a proven form of universal therapy, there would be no reason to restrict it to muscle or joint disorders, even if it involved some risk. But chiropractic use of manipulation in other illnesses contradicts much of the basic medical knowledge of the twentieth century. In such applications, no risk of injury is justified.

Unlike physicians, chiropractors receive little or no formal training in pharmacology and drug therapy. What they learn about drugs is often self-taught. That lack of scientific background or experience in drug therapy may well contribute to a dangerous approach to drugs by many chiropractors. Specifically, it involves undermining the use of accepted drug therapies and espousing the use of unproven ones.

Various chiropractic pamphlets for the public employ scare tactics against drugs. Such titles as "Drug-Caused Diseases" and "Drugs—Dangerous Whether Pushed or Prescribed" are typical. One published by the ACA in the mid-1970s, "Beware of Overuse of Drugs," lists scores of possible adverse reactions to such drugs as antibiotics, oral contraceptives, and medicines for high blood pressure. The pamphlet then asserts that chiropractors use no drugs, "thus avoiding drug-induced illnesses and dangerous side effects often more serious than the condition being treated." There's no mention that some of those drugs may be life-saving for patients who need them. The antidrug attitude can still be seen in a television cartoon released in 1989 by the ACA for use in elementary schools and viewed by a CU medical consultant. It states that "pills are old-fashioned" and advises a little girl in the story that she is a hypochondriac and should flush all pills down the toilet.

Chiropractic antipathy to medication, however, appears limited to prescription drugs—which chiropractors may not legally prescribe. Other medications, such as vitamin preparations, are widely recommended and sold in chiropractic practice. That distinction is potentially dangerous.

For the patient's safety, any prescriber (or critic) should have sufficient training to know when and why a specific drug is indicated. Chiropractors have no such training. Certainly, a course in nutrition at a chiropractic school is no substitute for years of training in drug therapy. Yet chiropractors sometimes presume they can treat complex illnesses with vitamin pills. This presumption is supported by at least a dozen companies that market "nutritional supplements" primarily or exclusively to chiropractors. Although the labels of these products usually don't say what they are for—thus avoiding the FDA definition of a drug (see Chapter 5)—"prescribing" information is provided by the manufacturers and their distributors through literature and seminars. For example, some companies issue product information sheets marked "restricted to professional use" which suggest that various concoctions can "nutritionally aid" eye conditions, kidney function, and many other ailments. In 1988 a *Consumer Reports* staff member managed to attend a seminar at which chiropractors received a manual describing how to prescribe a company's supplements for epilepsy, arteriosclerosis, and more than 100 other diseases and conditions.

A significant number of chiropractors—probably several thousand—practice what they call "applied kinesiology," a bizarre system of diagnosis and treatment based on the concept that every organ dysfunction is accompanied by a specific muscle weakness. Its practitioners also claim that nutritional deficiencies, allergies, and other adverse reactions to food substances can be detected by placing substances in the mouth so that the patient salivates. "Good" substances will make the muscles stronger, whereas "bad" ones will cause specific weaknesses. Treatment of muscles designated as "weak" may include special diets, food supplements, acupressure, or spinal manipulation. Critics have demonstrated that any apparent results of the muscle-testing procedures are due to patient suggestibility.

The number of chiropractors involved in dubious nutrition practices is unknown, but recent surveys suggest that it is substantial. In 1988, 74 percent of more than 2,000 chiropractors who responded to a questionnaire in a chiropractic newspaper reported using nutritional supplements in their practice. Typically they are sold to patients at two to three times what the chiropractor pays for them. Whether they are prescribed to "boost immunity," to combat serious disease, or just for "general good health," it is clear that there is no legitimate scientific basis for their use.

Another danger of chiropractic treatment, say its critics, is that it might divert the patient from seeking appropriate medical attention in time. The result, they contend, may have serious or even fatal consequences that might otherwise have been avoided. Little information is available about the frequency of such disasters, but court cases indicate that delays in proper treatment have resulted in mental retardation, paralysis, and death from tuberculosis, spinal meningitis, and cancer. In many of those cases the victims were young children.

Chiropractors have also been criticized severely for their overuse of X rays. X-ray films can, of course, show true bone abnormalities, such as fractures, tumors, and arthritic changes. Many chiropractors use them for this purpose, but some—who advocate X-ray examinations for all their patients—appear to use them more as a promotional gimmick than as a diagnostic aid. The use of X rays to detect "subluxations" serves no scientifically valid purpose and is unwarranted.

Some chiropractors still obtain 14″ × 36″ full-spine X-ray films on all or most of their patients. These films yield little or no diagnostic information but expose patients to unnecessary radiation. According to an analysis reported in 1986 in the *ACA Journal of Chiropractic*, a full-spine X-ray examination, used routinely as a screening device in a young adult, is twice as likely to cause a cancer as to detect one.

Politics Pays

Despite the dangers of unscientific treatment, chiropractors enjoy wider latitude in their scope of practice than any other health practitioners except physicians. By comparison, other independent health care providers must practice within far stricter limits. Dentists don't treat stomach ulcers. Psychologists don't order medication for a heart condition. Optometrists don't treat epilepsy. But chiropractors may get away with "treating" all three diseases by claiming they are caused by spinal problems. And they are permitted to offer treatment in "specialties" ranging from pediatrics to psychiatry—with little or no scientific training in any of them. Chiropractors have won that freedom without engaging in research or demonstrating professional capability in those fields. They have won it by one method alone: political action.

For years, grass roots politics has been the lifeblood of chiropractic. By marshaling the support of chiropractic patients, the profession has achieved an effective political voice in legislation affecting its licensure and services. And that voice has been its protection against science. Opponents of chiropractic come to legislative hearings armed with information, scientific studies, and official statements from national organizations. Chiropractors come armed with testimonials.

The inclusion of chiropractic services under Medicare, after a seven-year campaign by chiropractors and their supporters, provides a classic example. Against the combined opposition of the AMA, the U.S. Department of Health, Education, and Welfare, the National Council of Senior Citizens, and numerous other groups, the chiropractic lobby emphasized one primary weapon: the mailbox. Congressional aides were reportedly astonished over the sacks of pro-chiropractic mail that didn't seem to diminish. It got the message across.

In its long war with science, chiropractic has won most of the major battles. Since 1975 chiropractors have gained still more ground through antitrust suits filed against the AMA, several state medical societies, and other prominent health organizations. As a result of these suits—which cost millions of dollars to defend—medical organizations no longer discourage professional association with chiropractors, a few hospitals have admitted chiropractors to their staff, and many medical facilities are willing to perform laboratory tests or X-ray examinations ordered by chiropractors.

Ultimately, chiropractors seek inclusion as primary care providers under any future national health insurance program. In the past, the public's freedom to choose among health

practitioners has been honored in legislation affecting chiropractors—and it seems likely that this principle will be sustained if a national health insurance bill emerges. Before
chiropractic services are included, however, CU thinks that
public safety demands a searching review and thorough reform
of chiropractic practices by appropriate state and federal agencies.

Consumers Union's Advice

Overall, CU believes that chiropractic is still a significant hazard to many patients. Current licensing laws lend an aura of
legitimacy to unscientific practices and serve to protect chiropractors rather than the public. In effect, these laws allow
persons with limited qualifications to practice second-rate
medicine under another name. CU believes that the public
health would be better served if state and federal governments
used their licensing authority and their power of the purse to
restrict chiropractic more effectively. Specifically, licensing
laws and federal health insurance programs should restrict
chiropractic treatment to appropriate musculoskeletal complaints, limit chiropractic use of X rays, and ban all use of
nutritional supplements. Above all, CU would urge that chiropractors be prohibited from treating children, who do not
have the freedom to reject an unscientific therapy that their
parents may mistakenly turn to for help.

Rather than use the services of a chiropractor, CU thinks
it would be safer for people to consult other health professionals. Even when a patient is dissatisfied with a given physician's treatment of, say, a back problem, he or she can
consult another physician, such as an orthopedist, a physiatrist
(a specialist in physical medicine), a medical doctor who does

manipulation, or an osteopathic physician. Then, if manipulative treatment should be indicated, it could be performed by that practitioner or a physical therapist.

Despite this recommendation, some people will still decide to use the services of a chiropractor. For those who do, but who wish to minimize their chances of being victimized, CU suggests the following:

• Try to locate a chiropractor whose practice is limited to conservative care for musculoskeletal disorders, preferably a member of the National Association for Chiropractic Medicine.

• Avoid any practitioner who makes claims about cures, either orally or in advertising. Anyone who implies or promises guaranteed results from treatment should be held suspect.

• Beware of chiropractors who ask patients to sign a contract for services. A written agreement is not customary practice.

• Reject anyone who advertises free X-ray examinations or routinely uses full-spine X-ray films as a screening device. Radiation should not be used as a lure or gimmick.

• Don't make advance payments for a set number of adjustments. Most chiropractors have a flat office fee and don't offer discounts for prepayment. Nor is it accepted practice to charge extra for "units" of treatment, such as manipulation, heat therapy, and the like. These should be included in the office fee.

• Don't be pressured by scare tactics, such as threats of "irreversible damage" if treatment isn't begun promptly. And watch out for those who encourage "intensive" treatment because anything less would be a "patch-up job." The intensive treatment is more likely to apply to the patient's bank account.

• Reject any suggestion to have weekly or monthly check-ups for "preventative maintenance."

• Never buy vitamins, herbs, or other "food supplements" at a chiropractic office.

• Last but not least, check with a physician about the chiropractor's treatment plan.

12

The Overselling of Water Safety

Is household water fit to drink? People selling water filters and the like hope homeowners won't have the answer to that question. The less homeowners know about what might be lurking in their water, the easier it is for them to be sold on equipment they may not need for problems they may not have.

Companies in the water-treatment business could sell their hardware on its merits. Unfortunately, many companies have chosen instead to prey on the widespread fear that the water isn't safe to drink.

"Help Safeguard Your Future and Your Health," proclaims the headline on a glossy brochure for an osmosis "drinking water system." The system, says the brochure, "effectively reduces or removes contaminants found in many home water supplies, including sodium, lead, aluminum . . . *all of which may affect your health as well as the taste of your water.*"

An outfit in Virginia begins its brochure for a distiller this way: "The water in this country is getting so bad, it's disgusting. . . . Well, with the water THIS bad," the brochure goes on, only their distiller "is going to do the job. . . . The sooner you order one, the sooner you'll be drinking the PUREST water you ever tasted in your life."

A major water softener company adds this pitch: "We understand that a water improvement system is an investment in your family's well-being."

The home water-treatment business is still in its infancy, but it has attracted some 400 manufacturers, and sales are expected to top $1 billion a year by 1995. To move the merchandise, water-treatment sellers have to convince people that they have a problem. Some water is polluted, but most people don't have a problem with their drinking water, though they may not know that. So the sales pitches prey on fear or ignorance.

The Better Business Bureau says that inquiries about water-purification companies jumped 40 percent from 1987 to 1988. Inquiries don't necessarily equal ripoffs, but the BBB says many consumers have been stung. Merchandise doesn't do what was claimed, requests for refunds are not honored, and consumers are unable to reach companies to get service.

Granted, plenty of responsible businesses and salespeople are in the water-treatment business, offering products that live up to their advertising claims. Water softeners, for example, have been sold for years as a solution to scaly rings in the bathtub, deposits in the water heater, and anemic suds in the dishwater—and generally without exaggerated health claims. And any number of dealers sell water-treatment devices without resorting to deception. Indeed, when CU called several companies listed under "Water Softening & Conditioning Equipment, Service & Supplies" in the Yellow Pages to inquire about a reverse-osmosis filtering system, they all said they were willing to sell one, but that it probably wasn't needed if municipal water was being used.

But the safe-water purveyors aren't always so forthright. For example, a salesman recently contacted a CU staffer to try to sell him a battery of water softeners and such. The staffer listened to a one-hour pitch that included frequent allusions to unhealthy contaminants in the water. At one point, the salesman pulled out a sheaf of newspaper clippings about toxic-waste contamination in the area a few years ago. And he opened up a small kit of glass vials and chemicals to test the staffer's water on the spot. His test showed some sludge in the staffer's water.

The price for the ware: $3,500. The staffer said he'd like to think it over, but the salesman wanted a decision on the spot. (That can be one sign of a less-than-ethical sales pitch.) He may have feared CU's staffer would get an independent water test, which the staffer did. Result: the water was fine in every respect.

The Door-to-Door Sell

According to consumer-protection officials and victimized homeowners CU talked with across the United States, the sales pitch followed a common pattern. Some door-to-door sellers also try tactics like these:

• *The phony survey.* The salesperson claims to be taking a survey of water quality in the area. The homeowner may assume the salesperson represents a government agency.

• *The sludge test.* Once inside, the salesperson asks the homeowner to run some tap water into a bottle. The salesperson

adds a few drops of an unnamed chemical—probably a floc-
culating agent, which combines with dissolved minerals and
causes them to precipitate out of the water. A sludgelike
residue forms at the bottom of the bottle. The homeowner
is surprised. The salesperson looks concerned—but fails to
mention that the chemical visually exaggerates the amount
of minerals present, and that the minerals are probably not
harmful.

• *The washcloth test.* The homeowner is asked to get a clean
washcloth. The salesperson produces a container of "treated"
water and stuffs in the washcloth. Presto. Detergent dissolves
out of the washcloth and forms a layer of suds on the surface
of the water. The point of the hocus-pocus is to show how
the homeowner's "raw, untreated" water keeps the laundry
from getting clean. In fact, it's normal for garments to retain
some detergent when washed in unsoftened water. The detergent is harmless, and the test is meaningless. Further, "raw,
untreated water" is a complete mischaracterization for the 83
percent of the population served by a municipal water company.

• *The charts.* The salesperson produces charts that show
how the devices being sold remove 99 percent of various
contaminants. That may be true—when the unit is new, under ideal conditions, or if the unit is scrupulously maintained
by the owner. But the salesperson will probably not mention
that most of the "contaminants" are rarely found in drinking
water.

• *Bottles on the doorstep.* Someone leaves a small bottle at
the front door, with an official-looking note asking you to fill
the bottle with tap water so it can be tested. The results are
invariably the same: the water is "dangerously contaminated"
and should be treated with the company's product.

Too Much for Too Little

One of the more visible companies in the water-treatment business claims to have sold two million water filters, marketing them through a multilevel dealer network. CU's efforts to talk with company representatives were unsuccessful, but through the company's printed and video materials, interviews with former dealers, and information from government agencies, CU was able to get a picture of the way it operates.

The company sells by recruiting dealers, who become direct distributors when they sell $5,000 worth of filters in a month. The next level is sales coordinator, followed by national marketing director. At every step, the company offers bonuses for extra sales volume. And at every step, it encourages its people to sell to their friends, relatives, and neighbors. Put a filter in a friend's home for a week, the company suggests. It's the "puppy dog" approach—once someone gets used to having the filter around, it will be impossible to get rid of. Especially if it's being sold by a friend.

The promise of big payoffs tempts many; the company says it has 20,000 dealers. Dealers are told that with bonuses and promotions, their profit from the company's most popular model, selling for $179, can be more than $100. No wonder the company can afford to pay generous commissions to its sales force. Its training tapes include testimonials from dealers who are making six- and even seven-figure incomes. But some dealers have filed complaints charging that they were misled about the potential earnings and that they had to spend hundreds of dollars for filters they couldn't unload.

The filter that sells for $179 is less effective at removing contaminants than other filters CU tested that cost half as much. Whereas most units use inexpensive replaceable cartridges, the $179 filter must be thrown out once it has treated 1,000 to 2,000 gallons of water.

Some dealers claim that their devices are "approved by the Environmental Protection Agency (EPA)." The EPA doesn't approve or disapprove filters; it merely assigns registration numbers.

"Good News" Cards and Calls

The same tactics used to sell resort time-shares and vacation airfare packages are now being used to unload water-treatment hardware.

A congratulatory postcard is mailed out; it states that the recipient has been selected to receive one of five awards in return for calling to participate in a national promotion. The nature of the promotion is often not stated on the card. The prizes include such items as a car, $5,000 in cash, 100 shares of stock in a large company, a vacation for two in Mexico, and a pair of "Georgio Casini" diamond watches. Some outfits using the prize promotions dispense with the postcard and phone people directly.

Once the company has someone on the line, the salesperson begins a carefully scripted sales spiel like the following:

> You have been selected this year as a major credit
> card holder to receive one of five major awards worth
> up to thousands of dollars for participating in our
> nationwide pure water promotion. . . . I'm sure you
> are aware of the shocking deterioration of our na-
> tion's water supply, right?

The caller goes on to rhapsodize about the awards that await and gives a few details about the water-treatment device.

> We represent an appliance called an Activated Carbon water purification system. It's a regular kitchen appliance which is specifically designed to remove virtually all the chlorine and man-made chemicals in your tap water. . . . What we would ask you to do when you receive the unit is two quick tests. First, do a before and after taste test. Second, do a before and after test on your ice cubes. We know you will be shocked at the difference. And that is when you will realize just how important pure water really is!

The price for this unit is $598—double or triple the cost of the best carbon filters generally available. But then, *this* filter "includes the award, from the '89 Buick down to the $5,500 in cash . . ."

According to the Better Business Bureau, people will most likely be "awarded" a piece of costume jewelry worth a few dollars or a "vacation" for two that doesn't include airfare, meals, or other necessities.

Avoiding the Oversell

Homeowners should put their guard up if someone tries to sell them a water-treatment device they didn't know they needed. Have the water tested independently to find out whether there's a problem that needs to be corrected.

Other signals for caution: a salesperson who implies he or she is from the government; a salesperson who asks for a potential customer's credit-card number (unless the homeowner is familiar with the company); a salesperson who implies that the homeowner needs this device to protect his or her family.

Before doing business with any company they don't know, homeowners should call the local branch of their Better Business Bureau or consumer-protection agency to determine whether there are unresolved complaints against it.

Individuals with their own complaints can report them to their local Better Business Bureau and to the Federal Trade Commission (Washington, D.C. 20580). Information about water treatment is available from the Water Quality Association, a trade group, at 4151 Naperville Rd., Lisle, Illinois 60532.

13

Thirty-eight Ways
to Avoid Being Quacked

Many people think that quackery and health frauds are easy to spot. Often they are right. But quack promoters know how to appeal to every aspect of human vulnerability. Quacks offer solutions for every health problem, including some they themselves have invented. What sells is not the efficacy of their products or services but their ability to influence their audience.

How can a person tell the difference between reliable advice and a quack promotion? Here are 40 strategies to avoid being quacked:

1. *Remember that quackery seldom appears outlandish.* Don't make the mistake of thinking that quacks resemble the shady characters selling snake oil in Western movies. Quackery's modern promoters use scientific terms and quote (or misquote) from scientific references. Some actually have reputable scientific training but have gone astray. "Most successful quacks

now wear the white coat of science, the suit of the respectable businessperson, or the cloak of religion," says William T. Jarvis, Ph.D., president of the National Council Against Health Fraud.

2. *Ignore anyone who suggests that everyone needs to take vitamin supplements to be sure of getting enough.* Although some people might benefit by taking vitamin or mineral supplements, most people won't. During the past five years, the National Academy of Sciences, the U.S. Departments of Agriculture and of Health and Human Services, and the surgeon general have all issued major reports on diet and health which recommend that Americans get their nutrients from foods, not supplements. So anyone who suggests that *everyone* needs supplements should be considered an unreliable source of information.

3. *Ignore any practitioner who says that most diseases are caused by faulty nutrition or can be remedied by taking supplements.* Although some diseases are related to diet, most are not. Moreover, in most cases where diet actually is a factor in a person's health problem, the solution is not to take vitamins but to alter the diet.

4. *Avoid physicians who give vitamin B_{12} shots indiscriminately.* Periodic B_{12} injections are appropriate only when intestinal absorption of this vitamin is impaired—as happens in pernicious anemia. But some doctors prescribe them for a wide array of other conditions for which there is no proven benefit.

5. *Be wary of fad diagnoses.* Some practitioners seem to specialize in the diagnosis and treatment of problems considered rare or even nonexistent by responsible practitioners. Years ago hypothyroidism and adrenal insufficiency were in vogue. Today's "fad" diagnoses are "environmental illness," "candidiasis hypersensitivity," "hypoglycemia," and "mercury-amalgam toxicity." (Chronic fatigue syndrome,

while not rare, is also being overdiagnosed by fringe practitioners.) Be wary, too, of anyone who says that food allergies can cause a myriad of health problems. Claims of this type are being made by bogus nutritionists and a few hundred physicians who practice "clinical ecology." (These subjects are discussed in Chapters 3 and 6.)

6. *Don't trust anyone who claims that a single test can be used to determine the body's overall nutritional status.* Unscientific practitioners use a variety of gimmicks and gadgets as a basis for recommending supplements. One current favorite is hair analysis. For $25 to $40 plus a lock of hair, a person can receive a computerized report containing bizarre speculations about his or her health and recommendations for vitamins and minerals that are supposedly needed. Although hair analysis has limited value in the diagnosis of heavy metal poisoning, it is worthless as a screening device to detect nutritional problems. Other dubious tests—described in Appendix 2—include amino acid analysis, cytotoxic testing, live-cell analysis, and herbal crystallization analysis.

7. *Don't assume that all diplomas and other certificates in the health field are equally valid.* During the past few years, many unaccredited correspondence schools have been issuing "degrees" in nutrition and other health-related areas. Some require only the payment of a fee, whereas others require limited amounts of study—based on unscientific writings. The status of a school can be determined by checking with the state department of education, the U.S. secretary of education, or the Council on Postsecondary Accreditation. No unaccredited school offers reliable instruction in the field of health care.

Of course, the fact that credentials are reputable does not guarantee that their holders practice in a scientific and ethical manner. Even the medical and dental professions have a small percentage of quacks and charlatans. Nor does accreditation guarantee that a school's graduates practice rational health care. Accrediting agencies recognized by the U.S. secretary of education exist for both chiropractic and naturopathic schools despite the fact that many if not most of their graduates embrace unscientific concepts.

8. *Be wary of practitioners who describe themselves as "holistic."* Scientific practitioners regard holistic medicine as treatment of the "whole person," with attention to emotional factors as well as the person's life-style. But most practitioners who call themselves "holistic" use unscientific methods of diagnosis and treatment.

9. *Be wary of methods characterized as "alternative."* Chiropractic, homeopathy, naturopathy, acupuncture, iridology, reflexology, "nutritional medicine," and other dubious approaches are often promoted as "alternatives" to modern medical care. There are many situations in which a legitimate choice exists among effective treatments (for example, some health problems can be treated with either surgery or medication). But promoters of "alternative" methods have something else in mind. They consider scientific medical care as but one alternative among many, and tout the methods listed above as *generally* equivalent or superior to it.

Promoters of "alternative" methods often claim that their methods are "natural and nontoxic" and offer none of the complications of drugs and surgery. This ploy takes advantage of the fact that proven methods of treatment can have adverse effects. Some treatments described as "nontoxic" are nothing of the sort. For example, Laetrile, which contains cyanide, has poisoned people. But even if a treatment is "safe," it is hardly worth using if it doesn't work.

Some writers who promote quackery attempt to seem impartial by presenting "both sides" of a controversy so that their readers believe they can make a valid judgment. The information they present invariably is slanted to favor the quack method, but readers unfamiliar with the subject matter may find it difficult or impossible to detect this.

10. *Don't assume that all scientific-sounding health groups are respectable.* Unscientific practitioners often band together into groups that share their views. For example, proponents of chelation therapy have formed the American College of Advancement in Medicine, and advocates of "clinical ecology" belong to the American Academy of Environmental Medicine. (Clinical ecology and chelation therapy are discussed in Chapter 3.) Some groups have no membership requirement other than payment of a fee. Noteworthy among these is the American Association of Nutritional Consultants, which promotes a wide range of unproven "nutritional" practices. This group has even issued "professional member" certificates to household pets whose owners applied on their behalf.

11. *Be wary of any treatment method supported by a crusading group.* Promoters of unscientific treatment methods often encourage patients to lend political support through testimonials, letter writing, lobbying, and public demonstrations. A century ago, valid new ideas were hard to evaluate and were sometimes rejected by the medical community. But today, effective treatments are welcomed by scientific practitioners and do not need laypersons to crusade for them. Reputable voluntary organizations—such as the American Cancer Society, Arthritis Foundation, and National Multiple Sclerosis Society—have formed to work on virtually every important health problem. These groups support research and public education; they do not crusade for specific treatment methods.

12. *Don't fall for the slogan "freedom of choice."* Many promoters of unproven methods espouse a distorted concept of "freedom of choice" in health care. They state that consumers

should be free to purchase any type of health product or service without government interference. What they really want, however, is complete freedom for *sellers* to market their wares without proof that the products or services work—a situation that amounts to a license for quacks. Legitimate consumer advocates seek to balance the consumers' freedom of choice with requirements that providers be competent, honest, and accountable for unprofessional conduct.

The most aggressive group supporting the above concept of "freedom of choice" is the National Health Federation (NHF), which generates frequent letter-writing campaigns to support its political ends. The federation was founded in 1954 by Fred J. Hart, shortly after he was ordered by a U.S. District Court to stop distributing bogus electronic devices claimed to be effective for diagnosing and treating the gamut of diseases. Throughout its history, NFH has crusaded against government interference with unproven remedies or treatments. It has also opposed proven public health measures—smallpox vaccination, pasteurization of milk, polio vaccination, and fluoridation of drinking water supplies. A 1963 report released by the FDA stated, "From its inception, the federation has been a front for promoters of unproved remedies, eccentric theories and quackery."

In a comprehensive analysis issued in 1988, the American Council on Science and Health reached a similar conclusion. The council's report noted that more than a dozen past and present NHF leaders had been in legal difficulty for questionable health activities, and a few had even received prison sentences.

NHF's most notable political campaign spurred passage in the mid-1970s of a bill (described on page 213) amending the federal Food, Drug, and Cosmetic Act to reduce FDA regulation of vitamin products. Some members of Congress reported that they received more mail on this issue than they did about Watergate!

Another group lobbying for "freedom of choice" is the Coalition for Alternatives in Nutrition and Healthcare (CANAH), whose goal is a consitutional amendment that would enable anyone—licensed or not—to engage in any practice labeled "health care" so long as a single consumer wishes it to continue. Another is the People's Medical Society, which is antagonistic to the medical profession but uncritically promotes "alternative methods" in its publications. Organizations that promote unorthodox cancer treatments include Project Cure, the Cancer Control Society, the International Association of Cancer Victors and Friends, and the Foundation for Advancement in Cancer Therapy.

13. *Be wary of "faith healers."* Many charlatans take advantage of people's religious faith by claiming to have divine ability to heal people. Careful follow-up studies have never found evidence of a cure of an organic disease through faith healing. But many cases have been reported where people died because they trusted a healer and abandoned effective care.

The Faith Healers (1989), by magician James Randi, lays bare the trickery used by evangelistic healers who pretend to know about the medical problems of people in their audience whom they have never met. Most simply have confederates collect information by talking to the audience before the performance begins. In the case of Peter Popoff, who claimed to be getting the information directly from God, Randi actually intercepted radio transmissions from Mrs. Popoff backstage to a small receiver in Popoff's ear!

14. *Be wary of claims that weight can be lost without effort.* Diet quacks would like people to believe that special pills or food

combinations can produce safe, rapid, and permanent weight control. But the only way to lose weight is to burn off more calories than those eaten. To lose one pound a week, a person must consume an average of 500 fewer calories per day than he or she burns up. The most sensible diet for losing weight is one that is nutritionally balanced and aims for steady weight loss of one or two pounds a week. This requires self-discipline: eating less, exercising more, or preferably doing both. Most fad diets produce temporary weight reduction—as a result of calorie restriction and water loss. But they are invariably too monotonous and are sometimes too dangerous for long-term use. Unless eating habits are permanently changed, weight lost through dieting is likely to be regained.

15. *Don't assume that advertising is closely regulated.* Many newspapers, magazines, radio stations, and television stations make little effort to screen out fraudulent ads for health products or services. Even those that do may not be completely successful. Government agencies are able to stop some fraudulent promotions, but they don't have the resources to stop most of them.

16. *Base purchases of food and drug products on their ingredients, not the images or slogans used to promote them.* Ads for cold remedies, painkillers, and the like have one purpose: to induce sales. They can be deliberately vague and often are misleading. The best way to use nonprescription drugs is to learn which ingredient is effective against a given problem and to buy the product containing the ingredient and dosage required.

Ads for food products may not tell the whole story, either. "No cholesterol" products may be undesirably high in saturated fat (which increases blood cholesterol level), for example, or an ingredient touted on the label may be present only in insignificant amounts. Those who are concerned about what's in food should heed the ingredient list rather than the hype. And remember that what counts is overall diet, not some magic ingredient.

17. *Be wary of advertising hype.* News media may sometimes sensationalize legitimate medical breakthroughs in news reports as "amazing," "miraculous," or "revolutionary." But when words like these appear in advertising, the product involved is almost always a fake. One such product, Cho Low Tea, was marketed in 1989 with full-page ads in over 100 American newspapers. The ads stated that the tea "has kept Chinese slim for centuries" and was recently discovered to have "natural cholesterol-reducing properties . . . as effective as medically prescribed drugs in reducing cholesterol." More than 50,000 people placed orders totaling over $250,000 for the tea. It turned out, however, that not only were the claims false, but the tea itself did not exist. Its promoters had planned to repackage another company's tea with the Cho Low label but were arrested before they could do so.

18. *Be wary of claims made for mail-order health products.* These products are almost always fakes. Most mail-order health schemes attempt to exploit fears of being unattractive. Their promoters are usually "hit-and-run" artists who hope to make a profit before the U.S. Postal Service stops their false ads. Common scams include miracle weight-loss plans, spot-reducing devices (claimed to reduce specific parts of the body), blemish removers, antiaging products, baldness remedies, breast developers, and phony sex aids. Ads for these products often contain a money-back guarantee. But the guarantee is usually no better than the product. Contrary to what some people believe, the Postal Service does not license mail-order advertisers.

The most extensive study of mail-order health advertising ever published was done by the quackery committee of the Pennsylania Medical Society, which screened copies of 500 nationally circulated magazines during the summer of 1977 and found that about a quarter of them carried ads for mail-order health products. Altogether, about 150 products were advertised by 50 promoters. Not a single ad was judged legitimate by the committee.

The FTC has warned consumers to be aware that some television programs that look like talk shows are actually program-length commercials. Some programs of this type have promoted dubious weight-loss plans and food supplements. One tipoff, says the FTC, is that the product promoted during "commercial breaks" is related to the program's content.

19. *Be wary of anecdotes and testimonials.* Separating cause and effect from coincidence in health care can be difficult. So if someone claims to have been helped by an unorthodox remedy, consider—and possibly ask a physician—whether there might be another explanation. For instance, most single episodes of disease recover simply with the passage of time, and most chronic ailments have symptom-free periods. Some people who give testimonials have undergone effective treatment as well as unorthodox treatment, but give credit to the latter. Some people think they have been cured even though their disease is still active. Some testimonials are complete fabrications. A few have even appeared in the same issue of a newspaper as the testator's obituary!

Emil J Freireich, M.D., of the M.D. Anderson Hospital and Tumor Institute in Houston, Texas, has devised a tongue-in-cheek plan that could be followed by anyone wishing to become a successful quack:

A. Pick a disease that has natural variability.

B. Wait until the patient is going through a period when the disease has been getting progressively worse.

C. Apply the "treatment."

D. If the patient's condition improves or stabilizes, take credit for the improvement. Then stop the treatment or decrease the dosage.

E. If the patient's condition worsens, say that the dosage must be increased, that the treatment was stopped too soon and must be restarted, or that the patient didn't receive treatment long enough.

F. If the patient dies, say that the treatment was applied too late.

In sum, a good quack takes credit for any improvement but blames deterioration in the patient's condition on something else.

20. *Be suspicious of medical endorsements.* Companies marketing vitamins and other nutritional supplements sometimes claim that physicians or other medical scientists have endorsed their products. Some of these companies have even established "scientific advisory boards." Such companies often make false and illegal claims for their products. A striking example in modern times was United Sciences of America, a multilevel company that began selling food supplements in 1986 with the help of high-tech videotapes. The company claimed that its products would help prevent cancer and heart disease and that they had been designed and endorsed by a prominent 15-person scientific advisory board. However, of the seven most prominent "board members," six—including two Nobel prize winners—had neither developed nor endorsed the company's products.

21. *Don't assume that guests or hosts on radio or television shows are reliable sources of information.* Most talk show producers make little effort to determine the credibility of guests who discuss health topics. The area of greatest abuse is nutrition, where many more people are actively promoting misinformation than are opposing it. The sheer force of numbers works

against the truth. Remember, too, that it is legal for talk show guests to mislead their audience as long as they are not attempting to sell something at the same time.

22. *Don't fall for health food industry propaganda.* The health food industry would like people to believe that Americans are in great danger of being poisoned by additives and pesticides in foods and that soil depletion has robbed the food supply of vital nutrients. These ideas are used to promote the sale of "organically grown" and "natural" foods—at premium prices. But there is no reason to believe that foods marketed with these designations are any safer or are more nutritious than "ordinary" foods.

"Organic" foods are said to be grown without the use of pesticides or commercial fertilizers. From the plant's point of view, it makes no difference where its food comes from. Chemicals are absorbed by the plant in the same way regardless of whether the soil has been prepared with manure, compost, or manufactured fertilizer. Plants grow only if they receive enough nutrients, and their vitamin content is determined by their genes. Fertilizers can influence the mineral composition of plants, but these variations are rarely significant in the overall diet.

Although it is appropriate to be concerned about the possible abuse or overuse of agricultural chemicals, FDA market-basket studies indicate that pesticide residues are insignificant in the overall diet. Moreover, many studies comparing the pesticide content of "organically grown" and conventionally grown foods have found that their pesticide content is similar.

The word *natural* is said by its proponents to represent foods that are minimally processed and contain no artificial additives or preservatives. This definition implies that these substances pose a health risk. Actually, they help make the food supply safe, abundant, and palatable. It is illogical to condemn them with sweeping generalizations; the only proper way to evaluate them is individually.

Additives and preservatives make up less than 1 percent of food. Of some 2,800 substances intentionally added to foods, the most widely used are sugar, salt, and corn syrup—all found naturally. These three, plus citric acid (found naturally in oranges and lemons), baking soda, vegetable colors, mustard, and pepper account for 98 percent by weight of all food additives and preservatives used in the United States. Although one is occasionally found to pose a health hazard (sulfites, for example), the vast majority appear to be safe, and the overall level in the food supply should not be a cause for concern—or a reason to buy "natural" foods.

23. *Be wary of "antisugar" crusaders.* Another frequent target of the health food industry is sugar, which is accused of causing hypoglycemia, heart disease, and a long list of other health problems. The fact is, however, that when sugar is used in moderation as part of a balanced diet, it is perfectly safe. The only health problem related to sugar is tooth decay, which is increased by frequent consumption of carbohydrates that stick to the teeth. Proper brushing and flossing of the teeth plus adequate fluoride intake throughout childhood will minimize the incidence of tooth decay.

24. *Avoid publications that are loaded with ads for nutrition supplements.* Articles in such periodicals invariably make false or unproven claims for the ingredients of these products. Although such magazines and newspapers may also contain accurate information, separating fact from fiction can be difficult. Health food retailers—who get much of their information from these publications—are an equally poor source of information. Several large studies have shown that many retailers recom-

mend worthless supplement products instead of medical care for the treatment of serious diseases.

25. *Don't waste money on "health foods."* Although the term health food cannot actually be defined, it is still used to suggest that certain foods (usually sold at a higher price) have special health-giving properties not found in "ordinary" foods. Some "health" foods may indeed be rich in certain nutrients and thus can be a valuable part of a balanced diet. But no food has any special health-promoting property beyond those of the nutrients it contains. There is no logical reason to pay extra for a slogan.

26. *Be wary of pseudomedical jargon.* Instead of offering to treat your disease, some quacks will promise to "strengthen your system," "detoxify," "purify," or "rejuvenate" the body, "balance" its chemistry, release its "nerve energy," "bring it in harmony with nature," or correct supposed "weaknesses" of various organs. The use of concepts that are impossible to measure enables success to be claimed, even though nothing has actually been accomplished.

27. *Don't fall for paranoid accusations.* Promoters of dubious methods often claim that the establishment isn't willing to look at their evidence. They may even clamor for testing of their method. But if testing is carried out and their method found worthless, they charge that the test results are invalid because the investigators were biased or did not follow their methods exactly. This pattern of behavior has been prominently displayed by promoters of the quack cancer remedy Laetrile. During the late 1970s they mounted such a vigorous campaign that the National Cancer Institute agreed to sponsor a clinical trial comparing Laetrile to a placebo. During the planning stages, the proponents disagreed among themselves about various aspects of the study design. This ensured that no matter what was done, some of them could say the test

was done unfairly—which is exactly what they did when the test results proved negative.

Promoters of quackery often charge that the medical profession, the pharmaceutical industry, and the government are engaged in a conspiracy to suppress whatever product or service the promoters espouse. No evidence to support such a theory has ever been demonstrated.

28. *Forget about "secret cures."* True scientists do not keep their breakthroughs secret but share them as part of the process of scientific development. Quacks may keep their methods secret to prevent others from demonstrating that they don't work. No one who actually discovered a cure would have reason to keep it secret.

29. *Ignore anyone who promises to "strengthen" or "rebuild" the immune system.* The seriousness of AIDS has focused public attention on the immune system and generated all sorts of immunoquackery. Some promoters—including many who had previously claimed to cure cancer—promise an outright cure. But others appeal to the public at large by offering to boost immunity. Since nutrient deficiency lowers immunity, the quacks claim falsely that extra nutrients will increase immunity. The products involved are usually vitamin concoctions whose formulas are based on misinterpretations of scientific research. Claims that immunity can be boosted by psychological means should also be viewed with great skepticism.

30. *Don't buy "glandulars" or oral enzymes.* The idea behind these products is the primitive notion that they can strengthen or rejuvenate body processes that involve similar substances. "Glandulars" are ground up animal organs that supposedly can strengthen the corresponding part of the human body. For example, raw pancreas is given for the pancreas, raw heart for the heart, and so on. Enzymes such as superoxide dismutase (SOD) are pitched by reciting all the important func-

tions such enzymes play in the human body. But products of this type—which are proteins—can't actually reach the organs they are supposed to influence. Like other proteins, they are broken down into their component amino acids during the digestive process and don't enter the body intact.

31. *Be wary of herbal remedies.* Herbs are promoted primarily through literature based on hearsay, folklore, and tradition. Many claims are traceable to the writings of sixteenth- and seventeenth-century herbalists whose recommendations included herbs that contain cancer-causing compounds. As medical science developed, it became apparent that most herbs did not deserve good reputations, and of those that did (such as digitalis leaf for certain heart problems), most were replaced by synthetic compounds that are more effective. Many herbs contain hundreds or even thousands of chemicals that have not been completely cataloged. Although some might turn out to be useful, others could well prove toxic. With safe and effective treatment available, treatment with herbs rarely makes sense. Moreover, many of the conditions for which herbs are recommended are not suitable for self-treatment. "For all of these reasons," says Varro E. Tyler, Ph.D., former dean of Purdue University's School of Pharmacy, "consumers are less likely to receive good value for money spent in the field of herbal medicine than in almost any other."

32. *Be wary of homeopathic remedies.* Homeopathy is based on nineteenth-century theories that medical scientists consider nonsense. Despite this, homeopathic remedies are available from practitioners, health food stores, drugstores, multilevel companies, and a few manufacturers who sell directly to the public. Although remedies of this type can be legally marketed within certain FDA guidelines, the agency has never required proof that they are effective for their intended purposes. In addition, many "homeopathic" products

have been marketed with illegal therapeutic claims. (This subject is discussed in Chapter 3.)

33. *Be skeptical of any product claimed to be effective against a wide range of diseases—particularly serious ones.* There is no such thing as a panacea or cure-all. A few prescription drugs are effective against several different types of illnesses. But products claimed to cure everything are fakes.

34. *Ignore appeals to vanity.* One of quackery's most powerful appeals is the suggestion to "think for yourself" instead of following the collective wisdom of the scientific community. A similar appeal is the idea that although a remedy has not been proven to work for other people, it still might work for you. A third such motivator is the feeling of mastery that can result from taking an active role in one's own health care. Active participation can be very important to the success of legitimate treatment. Unfortunately, when a treatment regimen is bogus, the patient may enjoy a temporary feeling of accomplishment even while wasting time, money, and possibly his or her life.

35. *Adopt a healthy life-style.* Do whatever is reasonable to reduce the chances of becoming ill. To protect health: (1) don't use tobacco products; (2) eat a balanced diet; (3) maintain a reasonable weight; (4) exercise appropriately; (5) don't abuse alcohol; (6) wear a safety belt while driving; and (7) have at least one smoke detector in the home.

36. *Find a reliable primary physician.* The best way to take advantage of modern medical science is to establish a relationship with a trustworthy doctor—preferably before becoming ill. The best bet is a board-certified or board-eligible family practitioner or internist affiliated with a teaching hospital. Such a physician can steer patients toward high-quality medical care and away from frauds and quackery.

37. *Identify and use reliable publications.* Appendix 3 of this book lists excellent reference books and periodicals for a home health library.

38. *Don't let desperation cloud judgment.* When feeling that the physician isn't doing enough to help, or when wanting to put up a struggle against a condition diagnosed as incurable, don't stray from scientific health care in a desperate attempt to find a solution. Instead, discuss these feelings with the doctor and consider a consultation with another physician, preferably someone considered to be an authority in the field.

14

What Can Be Done?

The editors of Consumer Reports Books believe that the following measures will help reduce quackery's toll on society:

• The FDA, FTC, and U.S. Postal Service should attempt to develop better strategies to *deter* quackery and health frauds by making them less profitable. These strategies ought to include systems for earlier detection, quicker decisions to take action, and attempts to exact heavier penalties. Most important, the FDA should use more criminal prosecutions so that the marketing of products with false therapeutic claims can be deterred by the threat of imprisonment.

• The FDA, FTC, and Postal Service should be required to make meaningful data available so that legislators, news media representatives, consumer protection agencies, and the general public can understand what the agencies are doing about health frauds and quackery. This can be done by maintaining a list of prosecutions, both in progress and completed, that is accessible year-round through the agency's public information office and is published at least once a year in a report to Congress. The report should include tabulations of the number of health-related complaints received, the number judged valid, and the number subjected to regulatory action. The agencies should also be required to recommend improvements in the law that might enable them to work more effectively. These measures would enable legislators and the public to see the scope of the problem and what might be done about it.

• Federal laws should be passed to enable state attorneys general to prosecute cases in federal court so that the results are binding nationwide. This would correct the present situation where operators of a scheme prosecuted in one state can still continue it in the rest. It would also, in effect, greatly increase the regulatory resources available for consumer protection.

• The Postal Service and FDA should be given the same authority as the FTC to seek or negotiate large civil penalties against wrongdoers. The penalty could be equal to or greater than the profit from the scam. Currently, civil regulatory actions by these agencies carry no penalty unless the offender is violating a previous injunction or cease-and-desist order.

• The Proxmire Amendment to the Food, Drug, and Cosmetic Act ought to be repealed. This law, which was passed in 1976 after a vigorous campaign by the forces of organized quackery, weakened the FDA's power to police the food supplement marketplace. The agency can still attack products that are inherently toxic, but it cannot stop the marketing of useless products (such as rutin and bioflavonoids) for which no illegal therapeutic claims are made. Many such products are promoted with false claims made in books and magazines, where the author is protected by the First Amendment. Banning the products is probably the only way public protection can be achieved.

• The American Medical Association, which is by far the largest and wealthiest professional organization, should either reestablish its department of investigation and quackery committee or provide substantial financial support to independent antiquackery groups.

• Voluntary groups concerned with separate diseases should consider forming a liaison group to pool information on unethical and hazardous health promotions and report their findings to regulatory agencies, the media, and the public.

• State medical and osteopathic boards should systematically evaluate the work of physicians who engage in megavitamin therapy, clinical ecology, chelation therapy, homeopathy, "metabolic therapy," or other dubious practices to determine whether they are qualified to remain in practice. The penalties for practicing medicine without a license should be greatly increased.

• Dental boards ought to revoke the licenses of dentists who are inappropriately advising patients that mercury-amalgam fillings are toxic and should be removed.

• The FTC should issue a trade regulation rule identifying and banning false or unproven claims in chiropractic advertising.

• The FDA and FTC should rid the marketplace of "stress vitamins" and bogus "ergogenic aids." The United States should ban the sale of amino acids without a prescription, as Canada did in 1985.

• The FDA and FTC should rid the marketplace of nonprescription products whose names suggest properties that would not be legal to state on a product label or in advertising. This would include products falsely implied to improve a body function (e.g., *Brain Power Pack* and *Memory Booster)* or falsely implied to benefit an organ or body part (e.g., *Raw Adrenal* and *Vitamins for the Hair*).

• The FDA should require herbal products and homeopathic remedies to meet the same standards for safety and efficacy as drug products.

• The FDA ought to stop the illegal marketing of vitamin concoctions for the treatment of disease, as is currently done by manufacturers who sell most of their products through chiropractors.

• The FDA and FTC jointly should develop a consistent standard of substantiation for review of health claims for foods both on labels and in advertising. The FDA should then require preclearance of any label containing a health claim.

• Newspapers, magazines, and radio and television stations ought to develop and publish detailed advertising standards for screening out fraudulent ads for health products sold by mail. (Very few media outlets now have such standards.) The standards should include a provision that if a proposed mail-order ad is obviously fraudulent, it may be reported to an appropriate consumer protection agency. (That way, ethical media outlets can make it more difficult for bogus products to be marketed profitably through other media outlets.)

• State laws should be passed to define the practice of nutrition and restrict it to qualified professionals. It should also be made illegal to use the title "Doctor" or "Ph.D." without a doctoral degree from an accredited school.

What You Can Do

Even if the laws and the role of government agencies were substantially strengthened, consumer vigilance would still be needed. There are three main things you can do to protect yourself as well as others:

1. Learn the characteristic signs of quackery as illustrated throughout this book and summarized in Chapter 13.

2. Upon encountering any dubious product, service, or individual, check things out and complain to the appropriate authorities (see Appendix 1). Such action may save many people from being hurt and might even save someone's life.

3. Identify and use reliable sources of information. These should include health professionals, publications, government agencies, and professional and voluntary groups that deal with whatever health problems concern you. Hundreds of reliable agencies and organizations are identified in the 1989 edition of *Consumer Health—A Guide to Intelligent Decisions* and described in detail in the *Encyclopedia of Associations,* which is available in the reference department of most public libraries.

The following agencies and organizations are actively involved in combating health frauds and quackery. They can answer questions and may be able to provide pertinent literature either free of charge or at nominal cost. All of them appreciate being notified of questionable activity in their areas of special interest.

• The *National Council Against Health Fraud* is a 1,500-member network of physicians, registered dietitians, health educators, attorneys, government officials, and others interested in working actively against health frauds and quackery. It publishes a bimonthly newsletter, develops position papers, provides literature, and answers inquiries from individuals as well as the media. It also maintains a Task Force on Victim

Redress that offers help to individuals who believe they have been injured by an unscientific practitioner. Membership information can be obtained by contacting the council at P.O. Box 1276, Loma Linda, California 92340 (714-824-4690). Requests for victim assistance should be directed to Stephen Barrett, M.D., at P.O. Box 1747, Allentown, Pennsylvania 18105 (215-437-1795).

• The *Consumer Health Information Research Institute (CHIRI)* was established in 1989 to promote consumer and patient education activities, including studies of misinformation, fraud, and quackery. It maintains a publications list and can answer individual questions. Its address is 3521 Broadway, Kansas City, Missouri 64111 (816-753-8850).

• The *Arthritis Foundation* publishes reports and maintains a clearinghouse for information about arthritis treatment and arthritis quackery. Inquiries can be directed to local chapters or to its national office at P.O. Box 19000, Atlanta, Georgia 30326 (404-872-7100).

• The *American Cancer Society* has a committee on unproven methods, publishes many reports, and maintains a clearinghouse for information on questionable methods of cancer treatment. Inquiries can be directed to local chapters or to the main office at 1599 Clifton Road, N.E., Atlanta, Georgia 30329.

• The *American Dental Association* can answer public inquiries about questionable methods involving dental care. Its address is 211 East Chicago Avenue, Chicago, Illinois 60611 (312-440-2500).

• The *American Dietetic Association* can answer inquiries related to diet and nutrition quackery. It also maintains a QUEST file of case reports of individuals harmed by unqualified nutrition advice. For a copy of its annual "Good

Nutrition Reading List," send a stamped, self-addressed, business-size envelope to 216 West Jackson Blvd., Suite 800, Chicago, Illinois 60606 (312-899-0040).

• The *American Medical Association* issues reports related to unscientific methods through its Council on Scientific Affairs. For many years it maintained a committee on quackery and a department of investigation that kept track of dubious health activities, but these were abolished in 1975. The AMA still answers inquiries from the public, and its library contains recent quackery-related publications as well as archives from years ago. Inquiries should be directed to the AMA Public Information Department, 515 North State, Chicago, Illinois 60610 (312-464-5000).

• The *Candlelighters Childhood Cancer Foundation* can provide advice about questionable and unproven methods to families of children with cancer. Contact can be made by calling 800-366-2223 or by sending materials for assessment to 1312 18th Street, N.W., Suite 200, Washington, D.C. 20036.

• *Children's Healthcare Is a Legal Duty (CHILD)* is a nonprofit group working toward legal reforms to protect children from inappropriate treatment by faith healers. It maintains a victim registry and publishes a newsletter. Its address is P.O. Box 2604, Sioux City, Iowa 51106 (712-948-3295).

• The *Committee for the Scientific Investigation of Claims of the Paranormal (CSICOP)* conducts critical investigations of paranormal and fringe-science claims. It is composed of prominent scientists, educators, journalists, and technical consultants. It publishes a quarterly journal, *The Skeptical Inquirer,* and maintains subcommittees on astrology, paranormal health claims, and parapsychology. Its address is P.O. Box 229, Buffalo, New York 14215 (716-834-3222).

• The *Council of Better Business Bureaus* has worked with the

FDA to discourage media outlets from accepting misleading ads for health products. Its National Advertising Division, located at 845 Third Avenue, New York, New York 10017, receives and adjudicates complaints about nationally circulated advertising and sometimes persuades manufacturers to withdraw misleading ads. Local BBB offices sometimes can provide information or resolve complaints about health-related products or services; however, problems with licensed practitioners are usually referred to professional societies or state licensing boards.

• The *Federal Trade Commission*, Washington, D.C. 20580, publishes a few brochures about health fraud and is interested in receiving complaints about misrepresentations in advertising of health services and products (except for prescription drugs). Complaints should be addressed to its Bureau of Consumer Protection.

• The *U.S. Food and Drug Administration* publishes a monthly magazine, *FDA Consumer*, as well as many flyers and reprints pertaining to quackery. It also answers questions about food and drugs and can take regulatory action against products and devices that are unsafe or illegally marketed. Inquiries or complaints can be sent to its headquarters at 5600 Fishers Lane, Rockville, Maryland 20857, or to FDA district offices, which are listed under the Department of Health and Human Services in telephone directories for the cities in which they are located.

• The *U.S. Postal Service* is interested in receiving information about suspicious promotions in which the consumer is invited to send payment through the mail. Complaints can be sent through local postmasters or mailed to the Chief Postal Inspector, 475 L'Enfant Plaza, S.W., Washington, D.C. 20260.

Complaints to federal agencies may receive increased attention when a member of Congress is involved. So it is often a good idea to send a copy of a complaint to Congressional representatives or to ask them to make the complaint for you. Where more than one enforcement agency appears to have jurisdiction, it is best to complain to all of them.

Appendix I

WHERE TO SEEK HELP

Problem	Agencies to contact
False advertising	FTC Bureau of Consumer Protection Regional FTC office National Advertising Division, Council of Better Business Bureaus Editor or station manager of media outlet where ad appeared
Product marketed with false or misleading claims	Regional FDA office State attorney general State health department Local Better Business Bureau Congressional representatives
Bogus mail-order promotion	Chief postal inspector, U.S. Postal Service Editor or station manager of media outlet where ad appeared
Improper treatment by licensed practitioner	Local or state professional society (if practitioner is a member) Local hospital (if practitioner is a staff member) State licensing board National Council Against Health Fraud Task Force on Victim Redress
Improper treatment by unlicensed individual	Local district attorney State attorney general National Council Against Health Fraud Task Force on Victim Redress

| Advice needed about questionable product or service | National Council Against Health Fraud
Consumer Health Information Research Institute
Local, state, or national professional or voluntary health groups |

Note: See Chapter 14 for addresses.

Appendix 2

QUESTIONABLE PRACTICES AND PRODUCTS

Each of the following items has one or more of the following characteristics: (1) its rationale or underlying theory is inconsistent with accepted scientific beliefs; (2) it has not been demonstrated effective by well-designed studies; (3) its use involves fraud, deception, misinformation, or significant physical danger.

Acupressure (Shiatsu) A technique that uses finger pressure instead of needles at "acupuncture points."

Acupuncture A system of treatment purported to balance the body's "life force" by inserting needles into or beneath the skin at various points where imaginary horizontal and vertical lines ("meridians") meet on the surface of the body. These points are said to represent various internal organs. Although acupuncture can sometimes relieve pain, there is no evidence that it can influence the course of any organic disease.

Amino acid analysis of urine A procedure claimed by its proponents to be useful in uncovering a wide range of nutrition and metabolic disorders. As with hair analysis, the test report may be accompanied by a lengthy computer printout containing bizarre speculations about the patient's state of health.

Applied kinesiology A pseudoscience based on the belief that every organ dysfunction is accompanied by a specific muscle weakness. (*Note:* kinesiology, which is the study of the mechanics and anatomy of motion, is a legitimate science.)

Aromatherapy An approach based on the theory that massaging various plant oils into the skin or inhaling their odors can help heal hundreds of diseases and conditions.

Auriculotherapy   A variant of acupuncture based on the belief that the body is represented by various points on the ear. According to proponents, the arrangement corresponds to an inverted fetus, with the head near the earlobe. Proponents claim that acupuncturing specific sites on the ear can alleviate ailments that originated in "corresponding" parts of the body and that diagnosis can be performed by examining the ear for signs of tenderness or variations in electrical conductivity.

Autointoxication   A theory that stasis causes the contents of the intestines to putrefy, forming toxins that are absorbed and cause chronic poisoning of the body. This theory was popular around the turn of the century but was abandoned by the scientific community during the 1930s. No such "toxins" have ever been identified, and careful observations have shown that the bowel habits of individuals in good health can vary greatly.

Ayurvedic medicine   A set of practices promoted by some transcendental meditation (TM) organizations. Ayurveda (meaning "life knowledge") is said to be based on a traditional Indian approach that includes meditation, purification procedures, rejuvenation therapies, herbal and mineral preparations, exercises, and dietary advice based on "Ayurvedic body type." Proponents claim that "Maharishi Ayurveda eliminates disease at the source rather than working at the superficial level of symptoms. The goal . . . is to prevent disease and promote perfect health and longevity."

Bach flower remedies   Extracts of various flowers whose scents are claimed to restore health by correcting negative emotional states that underlie all disease. The method was developed by Edward Bach (1880–1936), a physician who practiced homeopathy.

Cellular therapy   Injections of animal cells into the human body, claimed by various proponents to cure disease, rejuvenate or "revitalize" the body, and prolong life. The cells are commonly obtained from freshly slaughtered sheep fetuses, but other animals can be used. The method is also called "cell therapy" and "live-cell therapy."

"Cellulite" removers   A variety of gadgets, creams, and potions claimed to remove the dimpled fat found on the thighs and buttocks of many women. "Cellulite" is not a medical term. Biopsies have shown that it is simply ordinary fatty tissue that bulges outward while the skin remains partially bound by fibers to the underlying tissues. (See also "Spot-reducing aids.")

Chelation therapy   A series of intravenous administrations of a synthetic amino acid (EDTA) plus various other substances (see Chapter 3).

Chiropractic   A broad spectrum of practices based on the false premise that most ailments are caused by spinal misalignments (see Chapter 11).

Clinical ecology   A pseudoscience based on the premise that multiple symptoms are triggered by hypersensitivity to common foods and chemicals (see Chapter 6).

Colonic irrigation   A "high colonic" enema performed by passing a rubber tube into the rectum for a distance of up to 20 or 30 inches. Warm water is pumped in and out through the tube, a few pints at a time, typically using 20 or more gallons. Some practitioners add herbs, coffee, or other substances to the water. Fatal infections have been transmitted with contaminated equipment. The procedure typically is recommended as a treatment for "autointoxication" (see above).

Complementary medicine   A term used by unscientific practitioners who claim to "integrate" both alternative and orthodox methods into their practice.

Cytotoxic testing   A bogus test purported to diagnose food allergies. It is performed by adding samples of the patient's blood plasma and white blood cells to samples of dried foods and examining them with a special microscope. The white cells are evaluated over a period of time to see whether they have changed their shape or disintegrated. Controlled tests have shown that the test is not reliable for determining allergies. When the New York State attorney general's office sent a sample of cow's blood to a cytotoxic laboratory, the lab reported that the "patient" was allergic to milk.

Electrodiagnosis   The use of a machine to diagnose "electromagnetic energy imbalances." Using a probe connected to the machine, the practitioner touches the patient's hands and feet and interprets numbers that appear on the computer screen. Devices of this sort are used by a few homeopaths and other practitioners to diagnose supposed allergies, vitamin deficiencies, and "degeneration" or "inflammation" of the body's organs (see Chapter 3).

Feingold diet   A diet based on the idea that salicylates and artificial food colors and flavors cause children to be hyperactive. Although many parents who have followed the diet have reported improvement in their children's behavior, controlled experiments have failed to support this hypothesis. Critics warn that it can be harmful to teach children that their behavior is determined by what they eat rather than by what they feel.

"Glandulars"   Raw glandular or organ tissues that have been dehydrated and processed at low temperatures to make tablets marketed as "dietary supplements." They contain no hormones but are claimed to "support" the corresponding organs within the body. Actually, the tissues—mostly proteins—must be digested before the body can absorb them, so taking the product simply adds insignificant amounts of amino acids to the body's pool.

Growth hormone releasers Amino acid supplements touted as aids in weight loss or sports nutrition. Claims for them are usually based on faulty extrapolation from experiments with animals. There is no evidence that these products, taken by mouth, actually release growth hormone in humans, produce weight loss, or enhance athletic ability.

Hair analysis A test misused by unscientific practitioners as the basis for diagnosing "mineral imbalances" or the presence of "toxic minerals." The test is usually obtained by sending a small amount of hair from the nape of the neck to a commercial laboratory for analysis. Most such laboratories issue computerized reports suggesting what supplements might be prescribed.

Herbal crystallization analysis A bogus test used as the basis for prescribing herbs. It is performed by adding a solution of copper chloride to a dried specimen of the patient's saliva on a slide. The resultant crystal patterns are then matched to those of dried herbs to determine supposed problem areas of the body and the herbs for treating them.

"Holistic" approach A slogan used mainly by unscientific practitioners. Scientific practitioners regard holistic medicine as treatment of the "whole person," with due attention to emotional factors as well as the person's life-style. But many practitioners who call themselves "holistic" use unscientific methods of diagnosis and treatment.

Homeopathy A system of treatment based on the idea that the symptoms of a disease can be cured by administering minuscule amounts of substances in undiluted concentrations, which would in healthy people produce similar symptoms of the disease. According to homeopathic theory, the tinier the dose, the more powerful it is (see Chapter 3).

Iridology A system of diagnosis based on the idea that each area of the body is represented by a corresponding area in the iris (pupil) of the eye. Physicians often gain valuable information about certain diseases by examining the interior of the eye with an ophthalmoscope, but iridologists claim to diagnose nutritional imbalances that can be treated with vitamins, minerals, herbs, and similar products.

Kirlian photography A method alleged by some faith healers to register their healing force ("aura") in photographs taken with a special apparatus. Critics have demonstrated that the nature of the pictures produced can be controlled by the degree of finger pressure applied to the apparatus and that the photographic images are also affected by perspiration.

Live-cell analysis A test performed by examining a drop of the patient's blood under a dark-field microscope to which a television monitor has been attached. Both practitioner and patient can then see blood cells and debris, which appear as dark bodies outlined in white. Proponents claim that the procedure is useful in diagnosing vitamin and mineral deficiencies, tendencies toward allergic reactions, liver weakness, and many other health problems that are treatable with food supplements. While videomicroscopy is a legitimate medical technique, live-cell analysis is useless in diagnosing most of the conditions its practitioners claim to treat.

Macrobiotic diet A restricted diet, high in whole grains, claimed by its proponents to improve health and prolong life. Proponents suggest that the diet is effective in preventing and treating cancer, AIDS, and various other serious diseases, but there is no evidence to support these claims. Although some versions of the macrobiotic diet contain adequate amounts of nutrients, others do not.

Mail-order diet pills   Various "miracle" products claimed to suppress appetite or alter metabolism. They include vitamin concoctions, "fat-burners," products claimed (falsely) to suppress appetite by filling up the stomach, and substances claimed (falsely) to block the absorption of sugar, starch, or fat. Ads for these products typically offer easy weight loss of a pound a day or more.

Metabolic therapy   A loosely defined treatment program that can include Laetrile, megadoses of vitamins, oral enzymes, pangamic acid, coffee enemas, and a low-protein diet (see Chapter 7).

Naprapathy   A variant of chiropractic based on the philosophy that contractions of the body's soft tissue cause illness by interfering with neurovascular function. Its proponents claim that gentle stretching of ligaments, muscles, and other connective tissue of the spine and joints of the body can restore health by relieving such interference. Naprapathic practice also includes nutritional, postural, and exercise counseling. Its practitioners are not licensed.

"Natural" food   A loosely defined term suggesting that a product has been minimally processed and contains no "artificial" additives.

Natural hygiene   A form of naturopathy that emphasizes fasting and food combining, a dietary practice based on the incorrect notion that certain food combinations can cause or correct ill health.

Naturopathy   A system of treatment based on the belief that the cause of disease is violation of nature's laws. Naturopaths believe that diseases are the body's effort to purify itself, and that cures result from enhancing the body's ability to do so. Naturopathic treatments can include "natural food" diets, vitamins, herbs, tissue minerals, cell salts, manipulation, massage, exercise, diathermy, colonic enemas, acupuncture, and homeopathy. Like some chiropractors, many naturopaths believe that virtually all diseases are within the scope of their practice. Naturopaths are licensed to practice in several states. In 1987, despite the unscientific nature of their beliefs, the U.S. secretary of education granted approval for an accrediting agency for naturopathic schools.

Nutripathy   A pseudoscience in which treatment with supplements and other measures is related to a formula devised by Cary Reams. Reams, a self-professed biophysicist, was prosecuted for practicing medicine without a license during the 1970s. Proponents claim that Reams's formula, derived from the results of nonstandard urine and saliva tests, reveals energy input and energy use within the body.

"Organic" food   A loosely defined term suggesting that the food has been grown without the use of pesticides or manufactured fertilizers.

Orthomolecular therapy   A treatment approach that utilizes large doses of vitamins, minerals, and various other substances normally found in the body. Also called megavitamin therapy (see Chapter 3).

Passive exercise   A purported method of weight control claimed to take the strain out of exercise by doing it for the individual. Offered at slenderizing salons, this approach typically involves a table that rocks or shakes or a motor-driven rowing machine or bicycle. Passive exercise may produce temporary relaxation, but it cannot cause weight loss. That requires *active* exercise in which calories are burned as a result of physical exertion.

Polarity therapy   A system of manipulation, stretching exercises, clear thinking, and diet claimed to restore health by removing blocks and restoring the flow of "life energy" between the positive (head) and negative (feet) poles of the body.

Psychic surgery   A procedure in which sleight-of-hand is used to create an illusion that patients can be cured with surgery that leaves no skin wound. Skilled observers have noted that animal parts or cotton wads soaked in betel juice (a red dye) were palmed and then exhibited as "diseased organs" supposedly removed from the patient's body.

Radionics and radiesthesia   Practices based on claims that electromagnetic forces emanating from nature can be detected with pendulums, dowsing rods, black boxes, and the like.

Raw milk   Milk in its natural (unpasteurized) state. Contaminated raw milk can be a source of harmful bacteria, such as those that cause dysentery and tuberculosis. "Certified" milk is unpasteurized milk with a bacteria count below a specified standard, but it can still contain significant numbers of disease-producing organisms. In 1987 the FDA banned the interstate sale of raw milk and raw milk products packaged for human consumption. In 1989 a California Superior Court judge ruled that Alta-Dena Certified Dairy and its affiliate Stueve's Natural must stop advertising that their raw milk products are safe and healthier than pasteurized milk and must label its products with a conspicuous warning. The dairy was also ordered to pay penalties of $123,000 plus $1.6 million in plaintiffs' attorney fees. The order resulted from a suit filed in 1985 by CU and the American Public Health Association.

Reflexology   A system of diagnosis and treatment based on the theory that pressing on certain areas of the hands or feet can help relieve pain and remove the cause of disease in other parts of the body.

Spot-reducing aids   A variety of products claimed to remove fat from parts of the body to which they are applied. These include vibrators, body wraps, and skin creams. Nothing applied to the outside of the body can reduce the fat content of the underlying body part. The only ways to accomplish this are through overall weight reduction or—in carefully selected cases—with plastic surgery such as liposuction. Exercise devices claimed to trim the abdomen, thighs, or arms are also dubious. Although exercise can tighten muscles in these areas, it cannot remove the fat between the muscles and the skin. For example, tennis players, who spend large amounts of time exercising only one arm, have equal amounts of fat in both arms.

Therapeutic touch   A system in which the hands are used to "direct human energies to help or heal someone who is ill." Proponents claim that healers can detect and correct "energy imbalances" by stroking the body or placing their hands above the afflicted part. Healing supposedly can result from a transfer of "excess energy" from healer to patient.

Tissue salts   A set of 12 products containing various homeopathic dilutions of inorganic minerals found in the body. Advocates of their use claim that the basic cause of disease is mineral deficiency, correction of which will enable the body to heal itself.

Appendix 3

RECOMMENDED READING

History of Quackery

Deutsch, R. *The New Nuts Among the Berries*. Bull Publishing, 1977. How nutrition nonsense captured America.

McNamara, B. *Step Right Up*. Doubleday, 1975. An illustrated history of the American medicine show.

Roth, J. *Health Purifiers and Their Enemies*. Prodist, 1977. An overview of the "natural health" movement and its critics.

Smith, R. L. *At Your Own Risk*. Pocket Books, 1969. A critical look at the history and shortcomings of chiropractic.

Young, J. H. *The Medical Messiahs*. Princeton University Press, 1967. A social history of health quackery in twentieth-century America.

Young, J. H. *The Toadstool Millionaires*. Princeton University Press, 1961. A social history of patent medicines in America before federal regulation.

Contemporary Quackery

Barrett, S. *The Health Robbers*. George F. Stickley, 1980. A comprehensive exposé of health frauds and quackery.

Barrett, S., and Casselith, B. R., eds. *Dubious Cancer Treatment*. American Cancer Society, Florida Division, 1990. A report on "alternative" methods and the practitioners and patients who use them.

Bennion, L. *Hypoglycemia: Fact or Fad?* Crown, 1985. A lucid analysis of the fad diagnosis versus the real disease.

Cornacchia, H., and Barrett, S. *Consumer Health—A Guide to*

Intelligent Decisions. Times Mirror/Mosby, 1989. A referenced textbook covering all aspects of health care.

Doyle, R. P. *The Medical Wars*. Prometheus Books, 1985. A lucid analysis of the scientific method and its application to 16 medical controversies.

Editors of Consumer Reports Books. *The New Medicine Show*. Consumer Reports Books, 1989. Consumers Union's practical guide to some everyday health problems and health products.

Fernandez-Madrid, F. *Treating Arthritis: Medicine, Myth, and Magic*. Insight Books, 1989. A penetrating analysis of arthritis quackery from ancient times to the present, plus up-to-date advice on scientific treatment.

Fried, J. *Vitamin Politics*. Prometheus Books, 1984. The classic investigation of megavitamin therapy and its proponents.

Gelband, H. *Unconventional Cancer Treatments*. U.S. Office of Technology Assessment, 1990. A detailed evaluation of dubious cancer treatments.

Gordon, H. *Channeling through the New Age—the Teachings of Shirley MacLaine and Other Gurus*. Prometheus Books, 1988. A critical look at mysticism, yoga, reincarnation, psychological techniques for "increased awareness," and many other components of the "New Age" movement.

Herbert, V., and Barrett, S. *Vitamins and "Health" Food—The Great American Hustle*. Lippincott, 1981. An investigative exposé of the health food industry.

Jerome, L. E. *Crystal Power—The Ultimate Placebo Effect*. Prometheus Books, 1988. Historical and scientific perspectives on crystal mythology.

Marshall, C. *Vitamins and Minerals: Help or Harm?* Lippincott, 1985. A comprehensive look at the sources, functions, benefits, dangers, and controversial aspects of vitamins and minerals.

Mirkin, G. *Getting Thin*. Little, Brown, 1983. Weight-control facts and fads.

Nolen, W. *Healing—A Doctor in Search of a Miracle*. Random House, 1974. A two-year study of prominent faith healers.

Randi, J. *The Faith Healers*. Prometheus Books, 1989. A devastating exposé of evangelistic faith healers.

Stalker, D., and Glymour, C. *Examining Holistic Medicine*. Prometheus Books, 1985. An exposé of "holistic" propaganda and practices.

Tyler, V. *The New Honest Herbal*. Lippincott, 1987. A referenced evaluation of more than 100 herbs and related substances.

Yetiv, J. *Popular Nutritional Practices: A Scientific Appraisal*. Popular Medicine Press, 1986. A referenced analysis of more than 100 nutrition topics of current concern.

Reference Books

Clayman, C. B., et al. *The American Medical Association Encyclopedia of Medicine*. Random House, 1989. A 1,184-page guide to over 5,000 medical terms, including symptoms, diseases, drugs, and treatments.

Fries, J. F. *Arthritis—A Comprehensive Guide to Understanding Your Arthritis*. Addison-Wesley, 1986. Facts about the causes and treatment of arthritis.

Herbert, V., and Supak-Sharpe, G., eds. *The Mount Sinai School of Medicine Complete Book of Nutrition*. St. Martin's Press, 1990. A comprehensive reference for nutrition facts and fallacies.

Lorig, K., and Fries, J. F. *The Arthritis Helpbook*. Addison-Wesley, 1986. A self-management program for coping with arthritis.

Pantell, R. H., Fries, J. F., and Vickery, D. *Taking Care of*

Your Child—A Parent's Guide to Medical Care. Addison-Wesley, 1984.

Renneker, M. *Understanding Cancer.* Bull Publishing, 1988. A guide to the causes, prevention, treatment, and psychosocial aspects of cancer.

United States Pharmacopeial Convention. *Drug Information for the Consumer.* Consumer Reports Books, 1990. A comprehensive guide to more than 5,000 prescription and over-the-counter drugs.

U.S. Preventive Services Task Force. *Guide to Clinical Preventive Services.* Williams and Wilkins, 1989. A detailed review of strategies for the prevention and detection of 60 illnesses and conditions.

Vickery, D., and Fries, J. F. *Take Care of Yourself—The Consumer's Guide to Medical Care.* Addison-Wesley, 1990. A practical manual with many flow sheets to help decide when medical care is needed.

Magazines

Consumer Reports, Box 53017, Boulder, Colorado 80321-3017.

FDA Consumer, Superintendent of Documents, Washington, D.C. 20402. Covers nutrition, food safety, drugs, and various other medical topics.

In Health (formerly *Hippocrates*), P.O. Box 56863, Boulder, Colorado 80322. Features well-researched articles about health issues.

The Skeptical Inquirer, Box 229, Buffalo, New York 14215. Features critical analyses of paranormal claims.

Newsletters

Consumer Reports Health Letter, Box 36356, Boulder, Colorado 80321.

Harvard Medical School Health Letter, P.O. Box 10943, Des Moines, Iowa 50340.

Healthline, Mosby-Year Book, Incorporated, 11830 Westline Industrial Drive, St. Louis, Missouri 63146.

The Johns Hopkins Medical Letter, Health after 50, P.O. Box 420179, Palm Coast, Florida 32142.

Mayo Clinic Health Letter, Rochester, Minnesota 55905.

Mayo Clinic Nutrition Letter, Rochester, Minnesota 55905.

Nutrition Forum, J. B. Lippincott Company, Downsville Pike, Route 3, Box 20-B, Hagerstown, Maryland 21740.

Tufts University Diet and Nutrition Letter, P.O. Box 57857, Boulder, Colorado 80322.

University of California, Berkeley Wellness Letter, P.O. Box 10922, Des Moines, Iowa 50340.

Index

239